HORMONES FOR "MORONS"

THE SCIENCE OF GRACEFUL AGING

MIKHAIL BERMAN, MD

Mikhail N. Berman, MD 8295 N. Military Trail, Ste G, Palm Beach Gardens, FL 33410

First printing 2021
ISBN 979-8-9851296-0-1 paperback
979-8-9851296-6-3 ePub
979-8-9851296-9-4 Kindle

Contents

Dedicated to Nahum Berman

Foreword

The late 1940s was a time when many young Soviet army physicians, not yet thirty years old, returned from the fronts of the Second World War. They were used to military discipline and hard work, and hardened by the adversities of the war, they were eager to advance in their careers during the newly arrived time of peace. Some of them quickly settled on their favorite area of medical or clinical research and were lucky enough to get positions in the leading medical institutions. Being of the same age group, with similar war experiences, they formed friendships with their colleagues.

N.N. Petrov Cancer Research Center in Leningrad (now Sankt Petersburg), the second largest Cancer center in the USSR, was no exception. A group of talented young World War II veteran doctors were writing their PhDs there. My father and Dr. Vladimir Dilman were a part of that group.

My father, Dr. Nahum Berman, worked in the Department of Urology.

His research was dedicated to the study of testicular cancer and the treatment of people affected by this disease. Needless to say, testicles are important endocrine glands.

His friend and co-worker, Dr. Dilman, was involved in the research of cancers of endocrine glands and endocrinology of cancers.

I remember Dr. Dilman visiting our house sometimes—for a dinner, or a party, or a cup of tea over which he and my father would discuss their work. Occasionally he asked me to show him a couple of guitar cords. He was trying to learn to play guitar.

Once, my father came home and laughingly declared to my mother, also a doctor, "Can you imagine, Volodya Dilman is studying why people age. Isn't it obvious that people get old because the time passes by?"

Later on, when I was already living in the United States, my father successfully operated on one of the regional Communist Party bosses. When asked what kind of gift he wanted for his successful treatment, my father asked to be allowed to visit me, his only son, in America. He brought with him a couple of books that were authored by his friends and gifted to him. In between those books was a book of Dr. Dilman, *Oncological Endocrinology*, in which he discussed his theory of aging. I did not pay attention and did not even open the book. I was busy studying for my medical licensing examinations to become a doctor in the US.

Father passed away shortly after arriving in the US, and I moved from Boston to Florida and began working as a family doctor.

In 2004, I was driving home from a medical lecture dedicated to the diseases of the thyroid gland, when my friend Vadim, Dr. Surikov, called me on the phone. As soon as he found out I was learning about the thyroid, he burst out in an enthusiastic diatribe about endocrinology. Vadim told me that he befriended an anti-aging physician, Dr. R., who got him interested in the interaction between the thyroid and adrenal glands, and that he had used this knowledge to successfully treat a multitude of patients.

When I came home, I looked for some medical literature on the topic, and it was then that I discovered Dilman's book waiting for me on my bookshelf. I opened it and looked through it.

That was when I learned about Dilman's theory of aging. He came up with the idea in 1954 and had formulated his theory by the late 1960s. The fact that he was my father's friend, and a person I knew well, made reading this book very personal.

Since that moment in 2004, I have dived into studying Anti-aging Medicine, attended multiple conferences, and read hundreds of articles. But it is Dilman's book, *The Grand Biological Clock*, that made me understand that almost all processes in the body are the result of hormonal actions, and they occur for specific reasons.

I've tried to get my friends to read Dilman's book—a book that I found as engaging as a suspense novel—but they would give up after reading a few pages, saying that it was written for doctors and not for lay people.

Ever since then, I have had the idea to write a popular book about the neuroendocrine theory of aging, but it is only now (many years later) that this project finally came to fruition.

Introduction

Nobody likes to get old. The dream of living forever has been in the human mind since time immemorial, and all efforts of medical science until now have been directed at increasing the length of life and postponing death. There is one problem with this approach. Prolonging life does not necessarily mean prolonging healthy, joyous, and productive life—and until very recently, it resulted merely in extending the stage of senescence, the condition or process of deterioration with age.

Modern medicine has achieved unprecedented results in prolonging the average life span for millions of people. Gone are the times when most people would die from infections at an early age. The biggest step toward a longer life span was the discovery of penicillin by Dr. Alexander Fleming in 1928 and the development of its commercial production by the pharmaceutical companies Lederle, Merck, Pfizer, Squibb, and Abbott Laboratories by 1944.

Between 1945 and 1950, the elimination of infections as a major cause of death led to a dramatic increase in life span.

Since then, due to further advancement of medical science, the world's average life expectancy has gone from 47 years in 1950, to 63.7 years in 1985, and to 73.2 in 2020.

Today in the United States, the average life expectancy at birth is 78.5 years, and in some countries—for example, Japan—it is close to 85 years.

This tremendous increase in life expectancy has led to a corresponding cardinal change in demographics, with the number of people in their seventh and eighth decades of life more than doubling since the 1950s. But do the majority of these people truly live in a state of health, as defined by the World Health Organization as "complete physical, mental and social well-being and not merely the absence of disease or infirmity"? Let us admit that most older people do not.

People do live longer, but they take multiple medications with innumerable (and often bothersome) side effects to postpone death. Many of them are lonely and depressed, often separated from loved ones, unable to care for themselves due to physical debility or dementia, relying on other people for basic functions and activities of daily living.

The major causes of death have shifted from infections and trauma to diseases associated with aging, such as atherosclerosis, heart disease, stroke, cancer, and diabetes.

From one point of view, it is very concerning that more people of advanced age are dying from just a few diseases than from the hundreds of other diseases known to medicine. But if we look at this fact from another angle, it is easier to find common features and origins if only a few diseases are involved.

There must be a reason why these diseases develop in the majority of aging people.

The name of this common reason is *aging.*

Therefore, the paradigm of medicine should change. We have succeeded in prolonging the average life span; now it is time to concentrate on extending the general state of health into the seventh and eighth decades of life and beyond, avoiding the development of debility, dementia, and dependency, which are characteristic of old age now.

Since the publication of the breakthrough book by Suzanne Somers, more and more people, women and men, are turning to *bioidentical hormone replacement therapy* to delay the symptoms of aging. Most of the popular books written about hormones talk about symptoms of hormone imbalances and how to treat them. They do not associate the phenomenon of aging with the natural and continuous pattern of hormonal changes in an organism.

Many processes are involved in aging, and it is impossible to separate one from another.

There are many theories of aging—wear and tear, thermodynamics, mutations, the Hayflick telomere aging-related theories, but what has caught my attention is the Regulatory Theory of Aging. It was formulated by the Russian doctor and scientist, professor of endocrinology, Vladimir Dilman in the late 1970s and early 1980s, and is undergoing a second wave of popularity in recent years.

He tried to explain why the process of aging and the diseases that appear with age are so similar in all people. He delineated nine normal diseases of aging. He explained how the stability of the internal environment could coexist with development and where the process of aging originates.

As an Anti-aging Physician, I see what a difference it makes to patient compliance when they receive explanations about processes in their bodies, the goals of the treatment, and ways to achieve these goals, instead of just instructions coming from a medical authority.

In other words, in order to do something well, a person needs to know why it has to be done and whether the results correspond to the goals he or she wants to achieve.

In this book, I have tried to describe and explain in popular terms the role of hormones in the process of development and aging, based on Dilman's regulatory theory, to enable thoughtful readers to make educated decisions about mitigating and postponing aging.

Chapter 1

The Body as a Society

If you look around, you will realize that we are living in a very complex society. 330 million people living together and working in unison, providing each other with food to eat, places to live, energy to utilize, transportation, construction, waste services, security, communications, border control, law enforcement, defense, and many other services.

For this sophisticated society to function smoothly and to guarantee the safe, peaceful, and productive existence of such a large number of citizens, it needs seamless interactions between different functions and services and requires and a centralized government to exercise tight control over these processes. A successful society cannot exist without an effective system of communications between members of the society and between members and the government. The evolution of society corresponded with the evolution of the way we communicate between ourselves, each development supporting the other.

With time, communications became more and more effective. While in prehistoric times we communicated through word of mouth, gossip, and personal meetings, societal evolution required more and more effective ways to transmit information between people. We went from communicating by messenger-delivered letters in ancient times and the Middle Ages, to postal service, newspapers, and magazines in the 18th century. The telegraph, the telephone, and the radio were invented around the second half of the 19th century. TV appeared just about 80 years ago. Now we are using satellites and the internet, and communication technology is the cutting edge of technological progress.

Human society can, in many ways, be compared to the society of cells.

Just like a society consists of its members, the body consists of cells. However, there are about 30 trillion cells in the human body—about 100,000 times the population of the US and 4,000 times the population of the world.

The body needs blueprints and regulations for building and construction (the genetic code). It needs a transportation system (the circulatory system) to move nutrients and oxygen into cells and waste from cells to the waste-processing facilities (the liver and kidneys).

It needs to be able to acquire energy (the digestive system) to run processes. It needs to have a border wall (the skin and mucosa) and to have a system of police and security (the immune system). It needs government (the brain) and intelligence gathering (the sense organs). And most importantly, it must have systems of communication (the endocrine and nervous systems) that connect every member to its neighbors and to the government.

Just as human societies mimic the way complex organisms work, so their developmental histories also share similarities. We can use society's development as an illustration to help us understand how and why life developed from simple single-celled organisms to complex multicellular ones.

In prehistoric times, our ancestors roamed the Earth as hunter-gatherers, looking for anything good to eat. They spent much of their time alone or with a small family group. Because the groups were small, each hunter-gatherer was occupied in the same daily activities: hunting and gathering whatever fruit, plants, fish, and animals they could find, catch, or kill.

Nearly all of them died in the jaws of predators, or in fights with other humanoids, or from infections or trauma. In other words, they died from external causes, and only a very few of them reached old age.

Of course, it is easier to survive with a larger number of members in the group, and family groups slowly but surely grew into larger tribes. Men were hunters and protectors and women kept fire and took care of children.

As technology advanced, tribes started to build cities, which had the advantage of offering better protection to their citizens. People had time to focus on a profession, and cities came to house large groups of people with the same occupations. There were carpenters and masons, tailors and shoemakers. They tended to live near each other.

Many old sections of cities still have streets named for the occupations of those who first lived there, like Blacksmith Street and Baker Street. Cities also had a government that promoted peaceful and lawful interaction between inhabitants. And each group—government, police, army, peasantry, artisans, craftsman, blacksmiths, and bakers— each group worked in unison to perform its function in the city.

The next stage was the development of nations, which had more sophistication and complexity than cities, including larger governments with more functions and better modes of communication. All these developments ultimately sought to achieve more safety and productivity for individual inhabitants, their cities, and the nation as a whole.

Human society progressed from family groups, to tribes, to cities, to nations, and this move toward larger groups with each member performing more specific functions is not that much different from the development of biological life from single-celled organisms to multicellular organisms of trillions of cells.

Eons ago, the simplest living organisms appeared on Earth. They consisted of one cell. They absorbed organic substances present in the water they inhabited, and they grew and subdivided. In effect, they were immortal. When a single cell grew to a certain size and had accumulated enough DNA and raw materials to make two cells, it subdivided into two daughter cells identical to itself—only smaller in size. Each of those cells then grew and, upon achieving a certain size and maturity, subdivided again. Theoretically, this process can go on and on, as long as there are enough nutrients for the cells to grow.

Such immortality has been studied in the laboratory, where scientists observed a strain of paramecium (a common single-celled organism that looks like a shoe) subdivide through 8400 generations. Paramecia are immortal, yet scientists have calculated that if single-celled organisms never die, then the progeny of a single paramecium would very soon exceed the volume of our planet Earth.

So why do single-cell organisms die?

They die if the conditions of their external environment change to the degree that they cause changes in their internal environment that are incompatible with life.

If the puddle where they lived has dried or frozen or overheated, if the chemical content of the water has changed, or if there are not enough nutrients for them to grow and subdivide, they will die. They are unable to adapt to these changes because of their simplicity.

In order to survive in the new conditions, they would need to undergo some kind of change, acquiring new properties and characteristics. Change takes time, and often, they do not have this time.

A good example of the process of changing properties is the development of antibiotic resistance in bacteria.

When exposed to an antibiotic, those bacteria that are not killed can change and develop an ability to destroy the antibiotic or to live in its presence. The bacteria that have undergone these changes will remain somewhat different from the original bacteria that were never exposed to the antibiotic.

The simplest organisms have very limited ability to adapt (adjust) to a change in external conditions. They die from external causes.

In principle, this is very much like how the early human hunter-gatherers died before reaching old age, from external causes (predators, disease, trauma). The simplicity of their society and technology did not give them much ability to adapt. Humans formed tribes to improve their chances of survival. In order to do this, members of the tribe needed to develop new ways to communicate and survive together.

It took nature millions of years, but eventually the unicells developed the same strategy. They started to congregate in small colonies for survival—just like the algae *Tetrabaena socialis*, the simplest multi-cellular organism discovered so far.

Tetrabaena socialis consists of four cells which are connected by microscopic tubules through which they communicate. They multiply by each cell dividing into four daughter cells which are connected from "birth".

This was a significant evolutionary change. They needed to undergo a change in individuality. Individuals stay together so the whole can operate at a higher level.

And just like humans learned how to communicate among themselves to act together, cells started to talk to each other by producing chemicals—and sensing chemicals emitted from nearby cells. These substances that send signals to nearby cells are called cytokines, which in Latin means "cell movers." The conglomerates of cells grew bigger and bigger, and became more and more sophisticated.

The next stage in the development of communications came with a need to send messages to cells located at a distance. These long-distance chemical signals are called hormones. Every multicellular organism has hormones—even plants.

Sponges are among the simplest of animals and consist of millions of cells. Their source of food is organic matter present in the water that flows through their bodies. They have no organs, but there are groups of cells that carry out different functions, conglomerates of cells arranged like ancient cities organized themselves by housing people of the same occupations close together. Sponges are so simple that they have never developed nervous tissue—yet, as primitive as they are, they have hormones.

This all comes from the evolutionary change from individuality to multicellularity. Individual cells remained together, sacrificing their individuality to become somewhat different individuals in a higher-level organism.

Sophisticated societies are much better at defending themselves against enemies. They have better and more technologically advanced armies and industry. This society has a faster and more efficient way to mobilize its resources in the time of war. And after defeating an enemy, they have a better ability to restore and return to a peaceful existence.

For human society, use of fire was probably the most fundamental step in the development of civilization. This was the first, the most basic way for humankind to use energy.

Fire was used to help prehistoric humans keep warm, to make food safer and easier to digest, to keep dangerous wild animals away. In other words, fire increased the ability of humankind to maintain the stability of the internal environment, exchange energy, and defend itself. The use of fire resulted in better chances for successful procreation and survival of offspring.

From this basic form of energy, just keeping a fire burning, humans progressed to using fire in making pottery, forging metals, sterilizing surgical instruments, and finally in creating motion. They made vehicles powered by fire and steam, then internal combustion, then electricity. The more society progresses, the more successful it becomes at obtaining and using energy to defend itself against enemies and improve the chances for its citizens to successfully procreate.

Sophisticated societies are better able to adapt, and the same is true for biology. It took nature hundreds of millions of years to invent the kind of creatures that were able to adapt to large changes in the external environment and defend themselves by actively normalizing their internal environment.

This higher level of adaptation required a much more complex organism consisting of many cells. The more complex an organism is, the better it can adapt, i.e., to actively respond to an unfriendly environment and return to its previous state.

For cells to work in unison for their protection, they too need organization. Organization is impossible without communications. Cells learned to send chemical signals to each other in close vicinity by cytokines, and at a greater distance with hormones.

Like the single cells, these complex organisms also ate, grew, and multiplied, but another basic requirement of life was attained: the ability to adjust or adapt to changes in the environment while maintaining the multicellular body's own properties. The more complex an organism is, the more ability it has to adjust to a changing external environment and survive.

There are 30 trillion cells that make up our body, organs, skin, hair, bones, and muscles, and they all work in unison, maintaining the system with complex communications between them. Different organs and tissues perform different functions and have different qualities. But every cell in the body has a way to communicate with her neighbors, and each one is also under central command control.

Remember that we all develop from one cell—the fertilized egg. So, how come the cells in our body look so different? A muscle does not look (or work) like a hair, neither does the skin look like an eye or a bone. But still, all the cells in the body were made from one single cell that divided many times.

Chapter 2

Three Basic Functions of the Living organism

Procreation

We instinctively distinguish living from non-living. We know from a very early age that living beings are not the same as non-living objects. Even for a small child, the difference between a frog and a stone is obvious. A frog is alive, a stone is not; a frog and a cat move, a stone and a cup do not.

From a biological point of view, living beings produce progeny, which are beings identical (or similar) to the parent. Bacteria, plants, mushrooms, and animals all procreate. They may use different mechanisms, but all living beings reproduce. Non-living objects do not.

A stone cannot produce another stone. A dead animal cannot bear offspring.

Every living organism consists of cells. Some of them, like bacteria or ameba, have only one cell. Others consist of trillions of cells, like humans. Every cell grows and accumulates building materials such as protein and fat within itself. After reaching maturation, a cell divides, producing two daughter cells identical to itself but smaller. Every cell reproduces in a similar manner. (Sex cells—eggs and sperms—do it somewhat differently by dividing chromosome pairs and splitting them between two daughter cells.)

Viruses represent a transitional stage between living and non-living nature. As soon as they are incorporated into a cell, they acquire the ability to procreate by hijacking the metabolic processes of the invaded cell, therefore becoming living beings.

However, when not inside the living cell, they are just very complex chemicals that are not representative of living nature because they do not have the capacity to reproduce.

Reproduction is the main difference between living and non-living nature.

Just like single-celled creatures need to grow and accumulate enough biological material to allow them to divide into two smaller cells, all complex organisms need to grow and mature to reach the stage of reproductive ability.

Energy production, growth of the body, and adaptation are needed to guarantee an ability to procreate, which is an ultimate goal of life, if life has a goal. Procreation ensures the continuation of the species. When an animal reaches the ability to procreate, it reaches the peak of its life. In effect, this is what it was born for.

After progeny is produced, nature acts as if it loses interest in an organism. The processes that created all the changes that occurred between conception and full reproductive development do not stop. An organism continues to develop, and if it lives long enough, these processes ultimately lead to diseases of aging and death.

A butterfly lives only one day, creates progeny, and dies. It is like there is a biological clock that determines the time of death of the insect.

The same can be demonstrated by such complex organisms as, for example, the Pacific salmon.

This fish is born in the upper reaches of rivers and spends its early life there, usually up to 2 to 3 years. When it becomes semi-mature, it travels from the river of its birth into the ocean. It lives in the ocean for 4 to 5 years, growing and developing and accumulating fat.

After reaching full maturity, it starts its final journey back to the river where it was born, sometimes several thousand miles away.

During this journey, the fish uses the fat accumulated throughout its lifetime to burn as energy. At the same time, cholesterol, which is synthesized from the fat, rises almost 10-fold. Cholesterol is necessary in large amounts for building the cell membranes of roe and sperms.

The salmon visibly ages during this journey. It grows "old" within 6 to 8 weeks. The jaws bend, the eyes sink in, the skin thins, and the immune system weakens. Massive physiological changes occur. The fish develops diabetes and atherosclerosis while cholesterol levels rise.

Finally, the salmon reaches the mouth of the river where it was born, and swims upstream to the exact place where it was spawned. There, it releases roe or sperms into the water, where conception takes place. After spawning is accomplished, every single fish dies. The causes of death are multiple infarctions of the heart, kidneys, brain, and lungs. By this time, the level of cholesterol in the blood has reached 1000 or more. The life cycle is completed, and the fish dies.

Salmon is a typical example of a semelparous animal. These animals put all available resources into maximizing reproduction. Semelparity is rare among animals but common among insects. Semelparous animals reproduce only once in their lifetime. After producing progeny, there is no reason for their existence because they have fulfilled their task. The biological clock has made a full circle.

Hormones produced by sex glands (ovaries and testicles) determine the sexual development of an animal during growth stages from embryo to fetus, to child, to adolescent, to adult. They are necessary to produce eggs and sperms. They regulate the mechanisms of copulation and processes of childbearing. They maintain the desire to procreate. However, sexual maturity does not occur until an animal achieves full size.

Energy Exchange

The second characteristic of living nature is the active exchange of energy between the body and the outside world.

Living organisms need to incorporate organic matter in order to produce energy inside their bodies to grow and survive. Without the influx of fuel, they cannot maintain the chemical reactions that continuously run inside their bodies and die, thereby becoming non-living nature. Non-living objects do not have this need.

All living organisms are open systems. They get fuel and building materials from outside of their bodies—they eat. Two opposite chemical processes are continuously running inside cells: catabolism and anabolism.

Catabolism is the breaking up of large, complex molecules and reducing them into water, carbon dioxide, and basic simple molecules. This process releases the chemical energy that is incorporated in their structure. Catabolism is similar to burning in that it releases the energy stored in large molecules. Catabolism supplies energy for two other functions of living: reproduction and adaptation.

Anabolism is the building of larger, more complex molecules from basic, simple building blocks, namely fatty acids and amino acids. These complex molecules are used to construct tissues and organs. Without this process, an organism will not be able to achieve sufficient size and maturity to reproduce.

The process of building more complex molecules from simple ones is called anabolism. In contrast with catabolism, it requires energy.

Living beings convert foodstuffs to energy by a series of chemical reactions. Just like burning fire releases energy in the form of light and heat, chemical processes in the body do this in the form of a special molecule called ATP (adenosine tri-phosphate). ATP is the energy currency of life.

As it is obvious from its name, ATP consists of the chemical adenosine to which three atoms of phosphorus are attached. It takes energy to attach the third phosphorus to ADP (adenosine di-phosphate), which already has two phosphorus atoms. Animals "burn" fats and sugars by a series of chemical reactions and use this energy to attach the third phosphorus atom to ADP, converting it into ATP. ATP then acts as a store of energy, like a microscopic battery. Energy stored in ATP is released when the third phosphorus atom separates, releasing energy used to attach it.

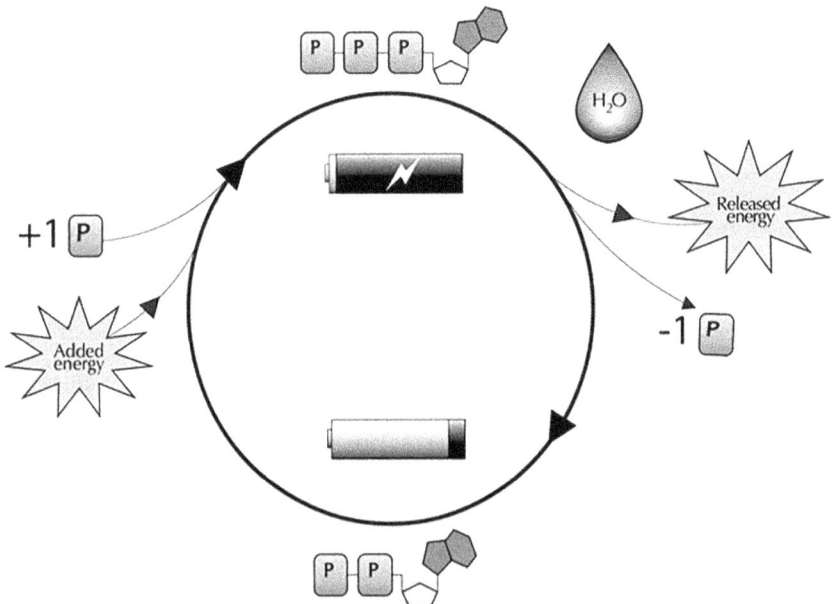

Fig 1. ATP: the energy currency of the body

The conversion of foodstuffs into energy can be done in 2 different ways: oxidation, which is *aerobic* (with oxygen); and fermentation, which is *anaerobic* (without oxygen). The fermentation process produces 18 times less energy than oxidation. This can be compared to the bellows that blows air into a blacksmith's forge, which raises the temperature by increasing the influx of oxygen.

There is a theory that the earliest organisms lived in an oxygen-poor environment and were therefore dependent on anaerobic ways of converting food to energy. They made only two molecules of ATP from each molecule of glucose. Later on, as a result of evolution, green plants that produced oxygen appeared, and the concentration of oxygen in the atmosphere increased. Many organisms were poisoned by such a high concentration of oxygen and died. However, some bacteria learned how to use oxygen in the burning process and began to produce energy in a more efficient way, making 18 times more energy from each molecule of glucose.

These bacteria apparently were internalized by other single-celled organisms and became mitochondria. Together, they formed a symbiosis (a mutually beneficial union) with the single-celled organisms, giving them the ability to utilize oxygen for efficient energy production in exchange for providing food and security for the mitochondria. Our body cells can still utilize anaerobic energy production but do it only when oxygen is in short supply.

We need the energy to maintain body temperature, build new cells, move muscles, run chemical processes, digest food, make hormones, maintain homeostasis, and all other functions of the body. It is interesting to note that the brain is the biggest energy consumer of all tissues. It makes up only 2.5% of the body but uses 10% of the body's energy.

If more food is internalized than is needed for survival, a surplus of fuel is stored as fat to be used when sources of energy are sparse. A very small amount of sugars—an immediate short-term energy supply—is stored in the liver and muscles in the form of animal starch (glycogen) for emergencies when the body needs a quick boost of energy.

The rate at which our body makes energy and runs other chemical reactions is regulated by the thyroid gland.

The utilization of fuels is regulated by the hormones insulin and growth hormone. We will discuss these hormones in detail later.

Adaptation

Life, just like non-living matter, is bound by several fundamental laws. Each law is required for the continuation of life, and none of them can be violated. The first fundamental law of life was postulated by the French physiologist Claude Bernard in 1865. It states: "Stability of the internal environment is the necessary condition of survival of an organism." The term homeostasis (*homeo* meaning "same", *stasis* meaning "state") was coined by Walter Cannon in 1926.

Conditions outside of our body constantly change. Weather can be cold or hot, food supply can be plenty or scarce, water can be abundant or deficient. Nevertheless, the chemical content of the minerals and nutrients in body fluids and body structures must remain within very tight limits. Better ability to maintain a stable internal environment in unfriendly circumstances increases chances of survival and thus chances of successful reproduction. The need for organisms to adapt to changing conditions is the main driver of evolution.

Single-celled organisms have a very limited capacity for adaptation due to their simplicity. This is why they can die if even a slight change in external conditions causes a change in their internal chemical conditions. In order to survive, they need to change their qualities and become different from their original form. A good example of this metamorphosis was mentioned in a previous chapter—the development of antibiotic resistance by bacteria. When exposed to an antibiotic, those bacteria that find a way to destroy the antibiotic or protect their cellular processes from its action manage to survive. However, those survivors become different from what they were prior to these changes.

Complex organisms gradually developed an ability to maintain their internal stability within tight parameters despite changes in the external environment. They developed mechanisms to defend themselves and to regulate the blood concentration of minerals and water, body temperature, presence of nutrients in blood and tissues, oxygen consumption, and other parameters, despite changes in outside conditions—and to return to the original state when the conditions normalize.

The greater the ability of an organism to maintain constancy of its internal environment, the more complex it must be. Specializing the cells into different organs was a gigantic step in the evolution of unicells into multicellular organisms, and all for the sake of increasing the capability of maintaining a stable internal environment despite external changes.

This ability to maintain homeostasis despite changes in the environment is called adaptation.

All evolution is a story of adaptation to unfriendly conditions by the development of new beneficial qualities. For example, adaptation enabled organisms to leave the water and live on the ground, just as others took to the sky. This transition was achieved by creating a stable water and mineral environment inside the body.

Amazingly enough, the liquids inside our bodies are almost identical to the water of the Cambrian ocean where life originated, around half a billion years ago.

If the ability to adapt is exceeded and an organism is unable to maintain internal stability, we call this a disease, which if untreated will lead to death.

Adaptation is regulated by the adrenal glands, which are located on top of the kidneys. This is why they are occasionally called *suprarenal* glands.

Let us see what materials make up such a sophisticated system that can exchange energy between the outside world and self, create self-like creatures, adapt, and survive an unfriendly environment.

Chapter 3

Body Composition

Four of the most important substances composing the body are water, proteins, fats, and carbohydrates.

The most abundant of these is water, making up 60% of body composition.

About 500 million years ago, all living beings lived in the water. To move out of the ocean, nature found a compromise to enable land-dwellers' cells to live in an environment of water, even though the organism itself was no longer surrounded by water.

The solution was to separate the "ocean water" surrounding their cells from the dry environment by building an impermeable border wall: the skin and mucosa.

This transition required a sophisticated system of regulation that could maintain constant concentrations of the various minerals inside their bodies, identical to their concentrations in ocean water. In effect, our cells did not leave the water and are still living in an ocean.

Proteins

Philosophically, life is described by Friedrich Engels as a "form of existence of proteins," which means that all life, at least as we know it on our planet, is based on protein. Without protein, there is no life.

Proteins are chemical substances made of chains of amino acids. Amino acids are small organic molecules that have nitrogen atoms in their structure.

Altogether there are 20 amino acids from which all proteins are made. Short chains consisting of 2 to 20 amino acids are called peptides (or oligopeptides, *oligo* meaning "few"), longer chains of amino acids (20 to 50) are called polypeptides, and the longest chains (50 to many thousands of amino acids) are called proteins.

Proteins are different in that they spontaneously fold up to make 3-dimensional structures depending on the order in which amino acids are connected in the chain. Proteins represent the qualitative transition from the linear world of sequences such as starches and fats to a 3-dimensional world of molecules that are capable of diverse activities.

Proteins differ from each other in the length of their chains and the order in which amino acids are connected to each other. There are more than 100,000 different proteins in the human body.

Proteins have several life-sustaining functions in the body.

The most important function of proteins is structural. They form a matrix that maintains the structure of the cells and everything in the whole body. Tissues such as bones, cartilage, ligaments, muscles, skin, and organs all have protein structures. If not for the structural properties of proteins, our body would be just a liquid solution of chemicals.

The second important function of proteins is transportation. Most substances are transported from place to place inside our bodies. A special group of proteins called albumins are responsible for the transportation of many substances. Albumins act as chaperones for other molecules, directing their travel to desired destinations and ensuring their delivery.

The third vital function is enzymatic. Enzymes are proteins that catalyze (speed up) chemical reactions in the body. Almost every reaction in the body requires the action of an enzyme to occur at the speed necessary to sustain life. Enzymes can speed up reactions by extreme amounts—for example, a reaction that takes a millisecond to occur in the presence of an enzyme might take millions of years without it. Like many catalysts, enzymes are not consumed in the reaction that they speed up.

In the body, there are more than 5,000 kinds of reactions, each of which is catalyzed by a specific enzyme. The substance that the enzyme is working on is called the substrate, the substance that is a result of a chemical reaction is called the product. For example, oxygen atoms cannot connect to molecules without the enzyme oxygenase, or disconnect without another enzyme, de-oxygenase. The enzyme hydrogenase attaches a hydrogen atom to a molecule, and dehydrogenase removes it. And so on.

This specificity of enzymes makes it possible to run reactions in the exact order necessary to maintain metabolic pathways—for example, converting foodstuffs into energy or building multiple steroid hormones from cholesterol.

The fourth vital function of proteins is defense.

The immune system produces special proteins called globulins. All the antibodies that protect us from viruses, bacteria, and other harmful invaders are made from globulins.

All proteins in the body are synthesized from amino acids, according to codes stored in the DNA. These codes are unique for each organism, and therefore, it is our genes that determine our specific protein content.

Fats

Fats are organic substances comprised of carbon, hydrogen, and oxygen atoms and are insoluble in water and oily or greasy to the touch. Fats are essential for life because they can form membranes to separate volumes of water. Imagine what happens if a drop of oil is dropped into water—it forms a fat bubble. Add another drop of oil, and it will make another bubble, but these two bubbles will not merge.

Most substances in the body are dissolved in water, and fats are the substances that keep us from being just a 150-pound bag of solution. They provide waterproof divisions inside the body.

All cell membranes (and the membranes of organelles inside the cells) are made of fatty substances and cholesterol. Membranes separate the water inside the cells from the water outside the cells.

Of course, cell membranes are not that simple. They are extremely sophisticated chemical machines that regulate the exchange of atoms and molecules between the extra- and intracellular environments. In fact, one world-renowned scientist has a theory of intelligent design based on the incredible complexity of cell membranes. He thinks that it is so complex of a structure that all history of life on earth is not long enough for cell membranes to evolve in such a short time.

So, the most important function of fats in the body is waterproofing, providing structure for cell membranes.

Aside from acting as cell membranes, fats have other essential functions.

Due to their energetic density, which is double that of sugars, they are used as a source of energy and a means of storing it.

As a source of energy, fats are responsible for maintaining body temperature as well as feeding muscle cells when they are not actively working. The ongoing chemical reactions of converting foodstuffs into energy and maintaining body temperature are dependent on the burning of fat. Fat deposits under the skin function as insulation, and fat deposits around some internal organs act as shock absorbers, protecting organs from trauma. At the same time, these fats are also functioning as energy storage.

Fats, in particular cholesterol, are the material from which all steroid hormones are made—testosterone, estrogens, progesterone, cortisol, aldosterone, and others. In all, around 40 different steroid hormones are made from minor alterations of the cholesterol molecule. So, we can say that without fat, the body cannot make steroid hormones.

Fats are essential for our breathing because they form a foam-like compound, surfactant, that keeps our lung alveoli inflated so that oxygen can be exchanged for carbon dioxide. A pack of balloons fits in your hand and has almost no surface area. But blow up the balloons and they will fill the room, with a hundred times the surface area they had before. This is what surfactant does for the alveoli—it keeps them inflated so air can reach the membranes, and it maximizes the surface area available for oxygen and carbon dioxide exchange. Fats significantly speed up the rate of oxygen transport in the lungs from air and into the blood.

Fats are soluble in other fats, and this is why fat-soluble vitamins A, D, and K, which are necessary for life, cannot be internalized without being dissolved in fat.

In order to be absorbed from the digestive system, fats need to be broken into microscopic droplets with the help of bile, and then broken down into simple fatty acids by the enzyme lipase in the duodenum. They are the hardest to digest of all three macronutrients.

Carbohydrates

Carbohydrates are substances made of carbon chains of different lengths with attached hydrogen and hydroxyl groups, where the proportion of hydrogen to oxygen is 2 to 1, as it is in water. Carbohydrates have important functions in the body, but they can be produced inside the body from fats and proteins.

The simplest carbohydrate molecules are called monosaccharides, the most abundant representative of which is glucose, which has six carbon atoms. When two monosaccharides are connected, they form disaccharides. Mono- and disaccharides are commonly referred to as sugars. Sucrose, the sugar that we use to sweeten foods, is the most common representative of disaccharides, consisting of one glucose and one fructose.

Plants produce glucose from water and carbon dioxide using the energy of sunlight.

Very long chains of carbohydrates are called polysaccharides. Two examples are starches and cellulose, the material used by plants for building cell walls.

Glucose is the most important energy source for all organisms. It is stored in the form of starches in plants, and as animal starch (glycogen) which is stored in small amounts in the muscles and liver for times when the body needs more energy than digestion or fat-burning is providing.

The carbohydrate ribose has five carbon atoms. It is a building block of RNA (ribonucleic acid—notice the word *ribo*), and DNA (deoxyribonucleic acid). Ribose is also a backbone of the ATP molecule, the energy currency of the body, and it is present in the coenzymes NAD and FAD, which are necessary for the electron transfer chain, an important part of the energy-producing mechanism.

Simple sugars such as glucose and fructose can be absorbed directly into the bloodstream—a very fast source of energy.

Table sugar (sucrose) is made of two molecules of simple sugars attached to each other. It takes a minimum amount of energy to break these two apart, so it can be absorbed even in the mouth. Starches are broken into simple sugars by an enzyme amylase that is present in the mouth, stomach, and duodenum. Their absorption begins in the mouth and continues throughout the digestive tract.

Another type of carbohydrate is cellulose, the structural part of plants. Cellulose is also composed of simple sugars, but our digestive tract lacks the enzymes needed to break the bonds between them, so we cannot obtain energy from it.

Even so, cellulose does play an important role in the body, as it provides nutrition for beneficial bacteria that live inside our gut. Cellulose also provides bulk which allows for food to pass faster through the digestive tract.

Chapter 4

The Neuroendocrine System

Not so long ago, the nervous and endocrine systems were seen as two separate signaling and regulating systems in the body—nervous being responsible for the physical messages, and endocrine being responsible for the chemical ones.

Today we do not see them as two independent systems but as one governing system with two ways of exercising control. The nervous system is fast, almost instantaneous, and uses electrical signals to send commands and receive reports. The endocrine system is slower and controls chemical processes in the body through chemical signaling and reporting. The electrical signals are called impulses; the chemical signals are the substances that we call hormones.

The nervous system consists of brain, spinal cord, and nerves. It controls muscles and some glands. It is also subdivided into the voluntary, or somatic, nervous system (the one we can control) and the involuntary, or autonomic, nervous system (which we cannot control). The somatic system realizes control of voluntary movements such as moving arms, legs, running, sitting, standing up, etc.

The autonomic nervous system works independently, controlling muscular activities that must run with strict order and regularity, unaffected by the state of our mind. This includes movement of bowels, breathing, heartbeat, and other functions we have no mental control over. The autonomic nervous system has two divisions: sympathetic and parasympathetic. Both control the same organs, but they exercise opposite actions.

The sympathetic system is the system of fight and flight. It accelerates the heart rate and breathing, slows the bowels, makes muscles tremble, etc. The parasympathetic system acts in the opposite way.

They oppose each other, but this allows for very effective control of processes, like the gas and brake pedals in a car. Just imagine driving a car without both pedals.

The nervous system consists of nerve cells, called neurons. Sensory neurons transmit signals from the sense organs on the periphery into the central nervous system (brain and spinal cord). Motor neurons transmit signals in the opposite direction, from the brain and spinal cord outward to the muscles and glands.

Each nerve cell has multiple appendages, called dendrites, which are connected to numerous nearby neurons and receive incoming signals from them. If the incoming signal is strong enough, it causes a chemical reaction inside a neuron that generates an electrical pulse. This signal is transmitted to another neuron through one outgoing filament, called an axon. Axons can reach up to 3 feet long in humans. An axon often branches and connects to the dendrites of multiple neurons.

It is important to understand that axons do not connect directly to dendrites to form electrical contacts. A synapse, a microscopic space, separates an axon from a dendrite. When an electrical signal arrives at the synapse, an axon releases a special substance, called a neurotransmitter, into the synaptic space. The neurotransmitter causes an impulse to be generated in the receiving neuron, and the signal can in turn be transmitted to another neuron or a muscular cell.

Numerous neurotransmitters are present in the nervous system. They are divided into two major groups: excitatory, which agitate neurons, and inhibitory, which calm them down. The effect of a neurotransmitter depends on the presence of corresponding receptors; almost like hormones. Some hormones—epinephrine, norepinephrine, and neurosteroids, also function as neurotransmitters.

It is extremely important to understand and remember the role of neurotransmitters in the nervous system because they play a big part in the process of development and aging in complex organisms.

The other system of control in the body is the endocrine part of the neuroendocrine system, which we will mostly talk about in this book.

The endocrine system regulates slowly occurring chemical processes inside cells such as basic metabolic rate, synthesis of proteins, growth and development of the body, and others. In the endocrine system, hormones may oppose the actions of other hormones, but these actions are not exact opposites as they are in the autonomic nervous system.

Both systems, nervous and endocrine, are vitally important, and without them the body would not be able to exist—just as organized society cannot exist without our systems of communication.

Both the autonomic nervous system and the endocrine system are controlled by a part of the brain called the hypothalamus, located at the base of the brain. The hypothalamus is the bridge between the nervous and endocrine systems, the organ where the two branches of the neuroendocrine system meet, the body's CEO, the CPU (in a computer, the Central Processing Unit is the part that reads a program's instructions and coordinates the flow of information to other components throughout the system).

Because the subject of this book is hormones, we will not get into the details of how the nervous system works, but we will concentrate instead on the endocrine system.

Chapter 5

Hierarchy

While hormones are the signals sent from glands to cells, these signals need to be received.

Until relatively recent times (the 20th century), we thought of a cell membrane as a little cholesterol sack containing some gel and organelles (little organs in the cell for making energy, growing, digesting, replication, etc.). Now we know that the cell membrane is more than just a little bubble made of cholesterol that separates cell contents from the outside environment. We understand that the cell membrane is a sophisticated system of communications between each individual cell and the organism as a whole.

The cell membrane has a myriad of small protein structures incorporated into it, which are called receptors. Like antennas, receptors receive chemical signals from the outside of a cell and transmit the signal inside to execute changes in cellular chemistry.

Each group of receptors responds only to specific signaling molecules, called ligands. Each ligand can attach only to its corresponding receptor to cause the specific desired effect. Every hormone, cytokine, neurotransmitter, growth factor, medication, and other substance has its own specific receptor.

Each group of cells has its own specific mix of receptors. This is why the signaling molecules (ligands) influence only those cells that have corresponding receptors—and not the other cells.

If this were not the case, all cells in the body would respond the same way to any signal sent from the brain, glands, or nearby cells, and what was intended to be a signal would just be noise. Instead, each cell in the body only responds to a hormone or other chemical messenger if it has the corresponding receptor.

The brain and glands are not the only sources of messengers that can influence cells. Cells themselves can influence and regulate receptors present in their membranes. They can increase or decrease the number of receptors and activate or deactivate them. This is a very important factor in understanding hormone sensitivity and resistance.

Our society is built hierarchically, with city, county, state, and federal levels taking care of different issues.

Nature invented a similar hierarchy to control complex organisms. Local groups of cells control each other by releasing cytokines. Tissues are controlled by hormones made in glands. Glands are regulated by releasing hormones from the "master gland," the pituitary, which in turn receives its instructions from the hypothalamus, the CPU of the body.

Cytokines, Local Control

Basic communications between cells are accomplished by substances called cytokines (*cyto* meaning "cell", *kine* meaning "move"). These are molecules that cells produce and release outside of their membranes. Cytokines, when released into the space between cells, send signals to other cells located nearby. This is how cells communicate between themselves. It is the most basic and ancient method of communication and is present even in primitive multicellular organisms.

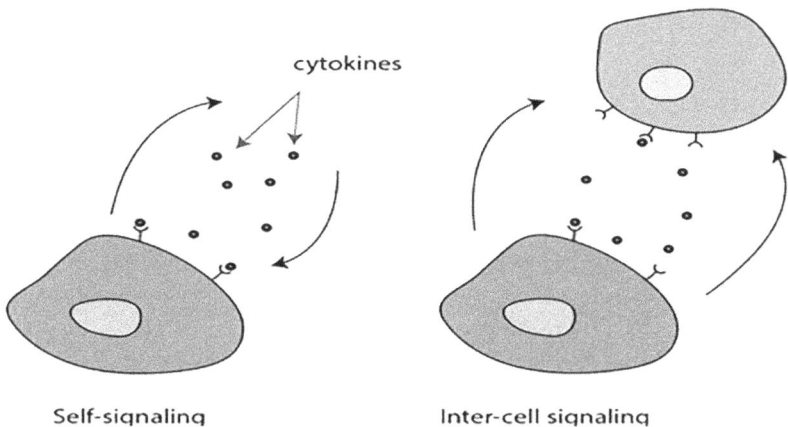

cytokines

Self-signaling   Inter-cell signaling

Fig 2: Cytokines: local control, self-control

Cytokines are especially important in the immune system. They balance the action of antibodies and immune cells. They also regulate the growth, maturation, and responsiveness of specific cell populations.

Hormones, Long-Distance Messengers

Hormones are produced in organs called endocrine glands.

Hormones are defined as substances that are released into the bloodstream from an endocrine gland to send a signal to cells located elsewhere, at a distance. For example, after a meal, the release of insulin from the pancreas (located next to the stomach) stimulates muscles and liver cells to take in glucose. The release of thyroid hormone from the thyroid gland at the base of the neck revs up the speed of chemical reactions in most cells of the body

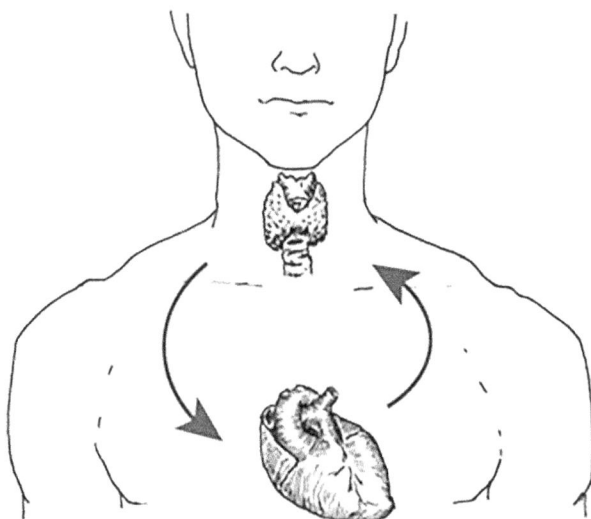

Fig 3: Hormones, control at a distance

Glands that are located outside of the skull are called peripheral glands.

The peripheral glands are as follows: the thyroid gland located in the base of the neck, the parathyroid glands near the thyroid gland, the adrenal glands (also called suprarenal glands) resting above the kidneys, the pancreas behind the stomach, the thymus behind the sternum, the ovaries in the pelvis, and the testicles in the scrotum. The activity (production of hormones) of each of the peripheral glands is controlled by a specific *stimulating hormone.* Stimulating hormones are produced in the pituitary gland, the "master gland."

Pituitary, the Master Gland

It is essential to know that glands do not release hormones at a steady rate. If that were the case, then it could not be considered a signal—it would be noise. Glands only release a hormone when they receive a command from the master gland, the pituitary.

The importance of the pituitary gland (or simply, the pituitary) cannot be overemphasized. Even its location in the body points to the importance of this organ. It is hidden at the bottom of the brain inside the skull, surrounded for protection by a special bony structure named the sella turcica (Turkish saddle) to protect it.

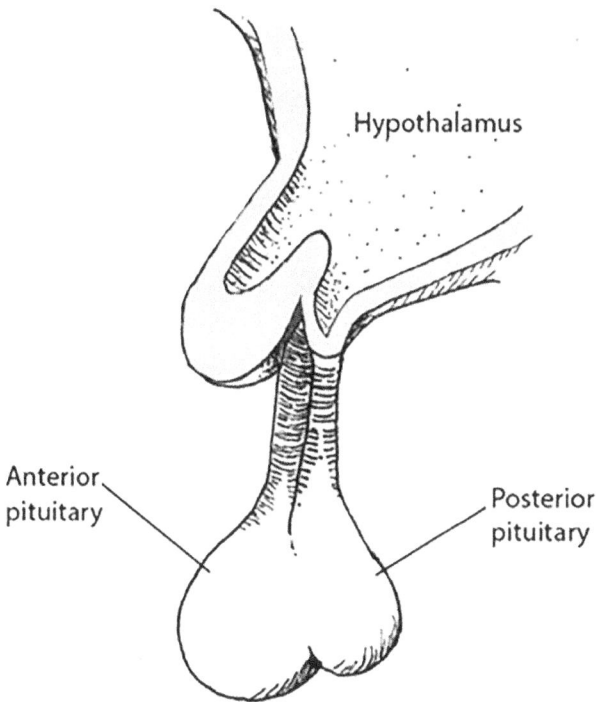

Fig. 4: Hypothalamus and Pituitary

The pituitary consists of two parts. One, located in the back, is the posterior lobe. It makes specific pituitary hormones such as anti-diuretic hormone, which regulates water content in the body by regulating the amount of urine produced, and oxytocin which is involved in uterine contractions, milk production, and some peculiar functions such as social interactions, trust, and love. The other part, the anterior lobe, is located in front of the posterior lobe, and it produces the stimulating hormones and growth hormone.

Stimulating hormones regulate the activity of peripheral glands: testicles, ovaries, adrenals, and thyroid, commanding the gland to increase production and release their corresponding hormones. This is why the pituitary is called the master gland. For each peripheral gland, there is a specific stimulating hormone.

The pituitary receives instructions from the main regulator of all unconscious processes in the body, the hypothalamus, and amplifies them to be heard by the peripheral glands. Upon receiving a command from the pituitary, peripheral glands release their hormones into the bloodstream. In order to receive commands from the hypothalamus, the pituitary has receptors to hypothalamic hormones.

The pituitary also has receptors for each of the peripheral hormones as well as its own hormones, thus enabling it to sense and participate in all three levels of negative feedback loops.

These are the main stimulating hormones produced in the pituitary:

Thyroid stimulating hormone (TSH) stimulates the release of thyroid hormone from the thyroid gland.

Adrenocorticotropic hormone (ACTH) stimulates the adrenal cortex to release the stress hormone cortisol.

Follicle-stimulating hormone (FSH) stimulates the production of eggs and sperms in sex glands

Luteinizing hormone (LH) stimulates the production of sex hormones in ovaries and testicles.

When the pituitary senses that a proper level of hormone has been achieved, the release of the stimulating hormone slows down, resulting in a decline of the release of the peripheral hormone. By measuring levels of stimulating hormone, we can determine if there is a lack or surplus of the peripheral hormone as interpreted by the hypothalamus.

But how does the pituitary know what gland to stimulate and when? The pituitary is just a gland. It does not have a connection to the outside world. It is, in essence, blind to the external environment. It can only respond to the signals it receives about levels of peripheral hormones.

However, organisms do not live in a vacuum. We need to respond not only to changes in the inside world, but to changes in the outside world too.

This leads us to an amazing structure located deep inside the brain, the hypothalamus.

The Hypothalamus—Where Glands and Brain Meet

We learn about external conditions through our sense organs—our eyes, skin, ears, nose, and tongue. These organs transmit information to the cortex of the brain. But it is not enough to just perceive a change in our environment, for example, a fall in outside temperature. To prevent us freezing to death, this information needs to be conveyed to the organs, which will increase heat production and decrease heat loss to raise body temperature.

The hypothalamus is the organ in the brain that can be compared to the CPU of the computer.

This organ-regulator receives the information from our sense organs about the outside world and from receptors inside the body about inside conditions. It analyses this information and then transmits commands to appropriate organs and cells to mount a response directed at maintaining homeostasis.

The hypothalamus is a part of the brain that controls processes in the body that need to occur automatically, continuously, and with strict regularity. These processes must be independent of the parts of the brain that regulate processes consciously. Otherwise, conscious parts of the nervous system might interfere with processes that must be performed in accordance with internal laws.

The hypothalamus functions independently from the central nervous system, obeying its own rhythm and signals from the body.

The hypothalamus controls not only the growth and development of the body (growth hormone) but sexual reproduction (sex hormones), temperature and speed of chemical reactions (thyroid hormone), adaptation (adrenal hormones), and utilization of energy (pancreatic hormones).

The hypothalamus and adjacent structures control pleasure and delight, sleep, emotions, appetite, heart rate and breathing, the functions of the digestive system, kidneys, and water and mineral metabolism.

It is a hybrid between a brain and a gland. It is where the nervous system merges with the endocrine.

The hypothalamus is a very special organ. On the one hand, it is a part of the brain consisting of nerve cells (neurons). It is connected to all parts of the central nervous system, so anything the nervous system knows about conditions inside and outside of the body can be rapidly transmitted to the hypothalamus. On the other hand, it is a gland capable of producing minuscule amounts of hormones, called *releasing factors*, that are sent to the pituitary to be amplified and transmitted to peripheral glands.

The hypothalamus converts rapid signals from the nervous system into slow but specific reactions of the endocrine system. One may ask, "Why do we need the pituitary gland if we have the hypothalamus to control glands?"

The answer is that it requires a large quantity of hormones to regulate endocrine glands all over the body, and the hypothalamus must be freed from this effort to be able to concentrate on its main job as a regulator. Essentially, the hypothalamic hormones act as the continuation of the nervous signals, ending in the pituitary. This design also allows the hypothalamus to switch to the next task immediately after transmitting instructions to the pituitary.

The hypothalamus is the main organ maintaining stability of the internal environment and controlling the growth and development of the organism.

The hypothalamus, in its turn, is controlled by the pineal gland that controls the body's circadian rhythm.

Chapter 6

Negative Feedback Mechanism

E very day you go to the bathroom. You do your business, flush the toilet, and probably never realize that you are using a cybernetic system that communicates with itself and controls itself using a negative feedback loop mechanism, just like your neuroendocrine system does.

It is based on the principle that if you want to achieve a goal, you need a signal from the goal to let you know when it has been achieved. When this signal is received, you can stop your action.

Nature invented the negative feedback loop hundreds of millions of years before human beings started using it, creating cybernetic systems of unsurpassed sophistication and precision. This fundamental cybernetic principle is utilized in biological, mechanical, electrical, and even social systems. It is the basis of all automation and self-regulation. How interesting it is that humans started designing negative feedback loops hundreds of years before it was discovered that nature has been using it all along in the regulation of processes of life.

But let's go back to the bathroom.

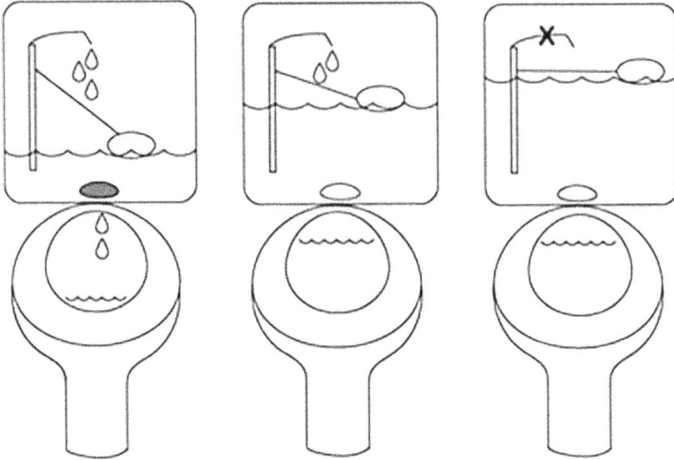

**Fig. 5 Negative feedback self-regulating system
maintains stable water level**

The water in the tank needs to be maintained at a certain level, be replaced when the level is low, and never be overfilled. Somehow, the system needs to know when to start adding water and when to stop adding water, so it does not overflow and spill on the floor.

This self-communication and self-control are accomplished using the float.

The float is connected to the source of water by an arm, and when the arm rises to the horizontal level, it plugs the pipe through which water is coming into the bowl. If the arm is below horizontal, the pipe is unplugged, allowing water to flow into the tank.

When you need to flush the toilet, you push the lever to elevate a stopper, which unseals an outflow opening on the bottom of the tank, allowing water to flow freely down to the bowl. As the water level in the tank drops, the float descends, pulling the arm down, which opens the inflow pipe and allows water to flow into the tank. When you release the lever, the outflow stopper seals the outflow opening, and the water level in the tank starts to rise. The float is raised by the rising water level in the tank and pulls the arm upward. You don't need to wait and stop the flow of water—as soon as there is enough water to elevate the float and raise the arm above horizontal, the inflow pipe gets plugged again, and the water stops. The tank is now prefilled for the next use, and water has not spilled on the floor. Water is maintained at a level sufficient to raise the arm to the horizontal position and no higher. If the outflow seal has a small leak, the water level will still be maintained, because as soon as the float descends, water flows in until the level rises enough to lift the float.

Negative feedback in the regulation of hormones is not as simple as the toilet system, but the principles are the same. It operates on not one—but three steps of regulation and three levels of negative feedback loops.

This three-level system is called the hypothalamo-pituitary-gland axis, where *gland* is the name of the peripheral endocrine gland being controlled.

There are several of them. For example,

1. *the hypothalamo-pituitary-thyroid axis,*
1. *the hypothalamo-pituitary-ovarian axis,*
1. *the hypothalamo-pituitary-adrenal axis, and so on.*

The hypothalamus is the part of the brain responsible for maintaining *homeostasis* (a steady state). If the hypothalamus detects any deviation from the steady state, it releases minuscule amounts of hormones, called *releasing hormones* (or *releasing factors*) that send signals to the pituitary gland to stimulate the appropriate release of hormones to stabilize the internal environment.

In response, the pituitary gland acts as an amplifier of the hypothalamic signal and releases the appropriate *stimulating hormones*, the ones that stimulate peripheral glands.

Both releasing factors and stimulating hormones are specific to particular peripheral glands and are named by the gland to which they relate. For example, thyrotropin releasing hormone (TRH) is released by the hypothalamus, thyroid stimulating hormone (TSH) is released by the pituitary gland, thyroid hormone is released by the thyroid gland, and other hormones follow the same pattern.

In the following diagram, we will call releasing hormone from the hypothalamus "Hormone #1", stimulating hormone from the pituitary "Hormone #2", and peripheral gland hormone "Hormone #3".

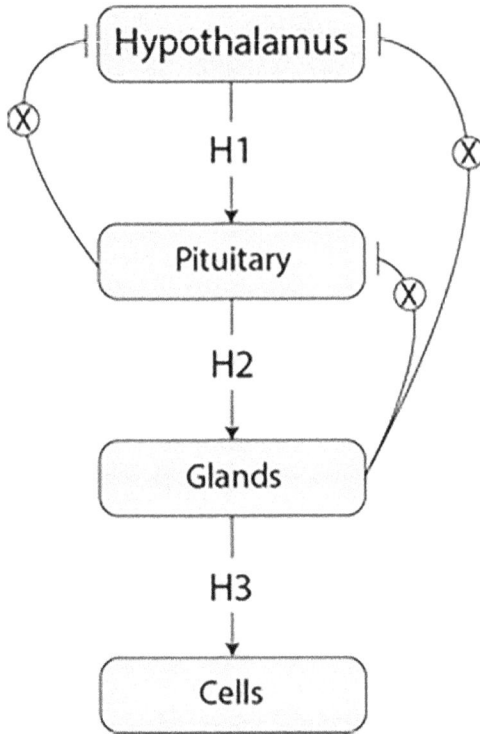

Fig. 6: Hypothalamo-Pituitary-Gland axis

When the hypothalamus detects that a level of Hormone #3 is too low, it produces releasing hormone (Hormone #1), commanding the pituitary to release specific stimulating hormone (Hormone #2), which stimulates the gland to release Hormone #3, raising its level in the blood.

The hypothalamus has receptors sensitive to Hormones below: #2 and #3.

The pituitary has receptors sensitive to Hormones #1 and below #3.

The peripheral gland has receptors sensitive to a Hormone above #2.

The raising of Hormones #2 and #3 to the optimal level is detected by the hypothalamus, which shuts off the release of Hormone #1.

The rise of Hormone #3 suppresses the pituitary gland from producing Hormone #2.

It is just like three toilet tanks in a row, is it not?

Chapter 7

How Do Hormones Work?

We know that hormones are chemicals that are produced at one place in the body and carried by the blood to distant sites of action, where they regulate the function of distant cells.

Here we need to be reminded about the protein structures called receptors. Receptors function as biological radio receivers. They receive and transduce signals in biological systems.

Each cell membrane, which is made of special fatty acids and cholesterol, has millions of protein molecules that are receptors. For example, an average cell membrane can house 10 to 20 thousand insulin receptors alone. These insulin receptors constitute only one ten-thousandth part of all protein on the membrane. As of now, hundreds of receptor types have been identified, but the work is far from done. Receptors are very specific and will only bind (connect) to a specific hormone. For example, insulin receptors will only bind to insulin and insulin-like growth factor 1 (IGF-1) but no other molecule. This quality is called specificity. They are also very selective—the insulin receptor will bind to a molecule of insulin in the presence of 100,000 other protein molecules.

Receptors can be located on the surface of the cell membrane. These are called cell surface receptors. They can be positioned with one part outside the cell and the other part inside the cell, in which case they are called trans-membrane receptors. Or they can be located entirely inside the cell, as intracellular receptors.

Hormones can only act through their specific receptors. A cell without a receptor for the hormone cannot respond to its action.

To say it another way, a hormone is a chemical signal, a molecule, that is sent from the gland to the cell. Only the cell that has specific receptors will respond to the action of the hormone, connect to the hormone molecule, and transduce its signal inside the cell.

Most hormones affect a few specific cells or tissues in the body. But there are few hormones that target most cells of the body: growth hormone, thyroid hormone, insulin, and cortisol.

The actions of hormones are very powerful, and that is why their levels are tightly regulated by a three-stage negative feedback mechanism originating in the brain, in the hypothalamus.

Even though levels of hormones are regulated by a negative feedback mechanism, receptors themselves are regulated too. The number of receptors can change depending on circumstances, and receptor molecules can be modified to regulate their activity.

The intracellular mechanism of action in response to the hormone can also be modulated to up- or downregulate the action of the hormone.

Endocrine hormones can be grouped into three different groups.

Steroids (the hormones constructed from cholesterol), which are sex hormones, adrenal hormones, and hormones derived from vitamin D.

Protein and peptide hormones like growth hormone, oxytocin, antidiuretic hormone, and others.

The third group is hormones derived from tyrosine, an amino acid. These are thyroid hormones, epinephrine, and norepinephrine.

Peptide and tyrosine-derived hormones are synthesized and kept inside the cells of the corresponding gland waiting for the signal to be released.

Steroids, on the other hand, are made on-demand from cholesterol and other precursors when an appropriate signal is received.

Protein and peptide hormones are water-soluble. Steroids that are derived from cholesterol are fats and cannot dissolve in water. The tyrosine-derived hormones epinephrine and norepinephrine are water-soluble, but thyroid hormones are not.

Hormones are transported in the blood in either bound or free form, depending on their water solubility.

Water-soluble hormones mostly travel unbound. Steroids and thyroid hormones, which are soluble in fat, are bound to carrier proteins, enabling them to be transported in the blood.

The binding of the steroid and thyroid hormones to a carrier protein, in addition, provides a circulating reserve of a hormone. It prevents hormones from escaping blood vessels and from being filtered out or metabolized by the liver and kidneys. It prolongs the release of the hormone into tissues. Thus, binding slows the onset and prolongs the duration of action of the hormone.

Changes caused by fat-soluble hormones (steroids and thyroid) begin slowly and take a long time to work. For example, thyroid hormones can be stored for several months and take several hours to several days to start acting, as opposed to epinephrine and norepinephrine, which start to be released within less than a second after stimulation and last for only 3 to 5 minutes before being eliminated.

Fat-based steroids and thyroid hormones easily diffuse through fatty cell membranes because fat dissolves in fat. As a result, their receptors are located inside the cell in the cytoplasm or nucleus. In most cases, fat-soluble hormones that make their way to the nucleus affect the DNA or RNA to activate or inhibit genes.

Water-soluble hormones, on the other hand, cannot penetrate through the fatty cell membrane and thus can only affect receptors located on or within the cell membrane. Their action usually results in the opening of channels in the membrane or the formation of a complex with another receptor, which in turn causes the creation of a so-called second messenger (the hormone being the "first" messenger), a molecule that transduces signals within the cell to change the cell's chemistry. Usually, the second messenger is the sugar-derived molecule called cyclic adenosine-monophosphate (cAMP), a cousin of ATP, the energy molecule.

Hormones are usually regulated by negative feedback. Receptors themselves can also be regulated. The most common scenario is the downregulation of receptors. The process of downregulation begins when the hormone binds to its specific receptor and starts a series of reactions inside the cell. Unbound copies of the same receptor are removed or deactivated until after the action of the hormone has been completed.

Hormones that have done their work get eliminated in three ways. They can be taken up and used inside the target cell, they can be metabolized and excreted by kidneys in the urine, or they can be metabolized by the liver and excreted into the bowel. Once in the bowel, they may be converted to active hormones by gut bacteria and reabsorbed back into the bloodstream.

Chapter 8

The History of Aging

Aging is not a purely human phenomenon. It happens throughout the animal kingdom. But in contrast with humans, most animals do not live long enough to achieve old age. If they are lucky enough to achieve the reproductive stage, they have a short time to bear progeny. As soon as aging starts and an animal becomes weaker and slower, its capacity to obtain food and mates declines, and it succumbs to competitors, predators, or hunger. Therefore, even if aging is not a purely human phenomenon, because of the advancement of society, only humans have a chance to live past the first symptoms of age-related functional decline. Even now, there are tribes on Earth that sentence aging persons to die when they lose their ability to provide for themselves. The act of observing aging, and the gradual decline that accompanies it, made humans dream of escaping this destiny.

From time immemorial, since the appearance of society, humans have dreamed of extending their life span. In Sumerian documents dating to 4000 years ago, in *The Epic of Gilgamesh*, Gilgamesh is a hero who goes on a quest to find eternal life, and fails to find it.

Ponce de León went on his journey to America to find the Fountain of Youth—and also failed.

Throughout human history, scientists have attempted to find the cause of aging, and the theories explaining this process changed as science and technology advanced.

When the laws of physics, especially the Newtonian laws, were discovered, and all processes in the universe seemed to abide by these laws, major technological advances were made.

The organism (from the point of view of these laws) looked like a well-designed machine, though extremely complex. The process of aging was attributed to wear and tear of parts of the body, just as machines break down after prolonged use due to fatigue of the metals they are made from.

After a while, scientific discoveries were made about the nature of energy. The laws of thermodynamics were formulated. They were used to explain the process of aging based on the law of the gradual increase of entropy, which limits the time span of every system in the universe. Nothing lasts forever.

The energy theory of aging was based on the fact that the ratio of energy used by an organism (measured in calories per gram per day) is more or less constant for complex organisms. Small animals, whose ratio of surface area to body mass is higher than in larger animals, live shorter lives because of greater heat loss, therefore requiring more energy.

Since living organisms are open systems and are able to procure energy from the environment, this theory cannot explain how disturbances in the environment cause changes in living organisms, distinguishing them from other natural forms of nature.

Later on, advances in genetics revealed that all mechanisms of life in a cell are determined by DNA. Changes to genes are called mutations. They play a significant role in the evolution of living nature, but damage to DNA from chemical and physical factors such as free radicals, radiation, and toxins may lead to harmful mutations, and these were thought of as a major reason for aging.

In these theories, the harmful mutations, or changes in genetic code, were considered as causing chaos in the functions of the body. As time passes, mutations and errors accumulate and lead to malfunctions, resulting in death.

Mutations and accumulation of errors may contribute to the mechanism of aging, but complex organisms actually have the ability to repair damaged DNA. The question, therefore, arises—why do these mechanisms become less efficient over a lifetime?

A theory of aging developed by Leonard Hayflick may shine some light on this.

The Hayflick Limit establishes the maximum number of divisions a cell is capable of in each species. At both ends of every chromosome, there are regions of DNA called telomeres which become shorter with every division of the cell. When these telomeres reach a certain length, the cell commits suicide, a process called apoptosis. Telomeres may be damaged or shortened by external factors in addition to the division itself. Thus, according to this theory, aging is a process of gradual loss of ability of cells to divide. However, this theory cannot explain why processes of aging in most higher organisms are so similar and universal.

There is also a group of theories of aging based on a systemic approach, or assessing an organism as a whole, which is based on cybernetics, a system of control and communications in self-regulating systems. These theories, which simply apply principles of cybernetics to a complex living organism, do not explain the role of the neuroendocrine system in the process of aging because there is no explanation of why it gradually fails to accomplish its principal task of maintaining homeostasis.

While none of these theories are perfect, each of them does manage to explain a different aspect of aging.

Mechanical theory can be easily seen in the wear and tear of our joints, especially when the ability of the body to repair itself diminishes with age.

The energy theory can explain the increasing inefficiency of energy use and production.

The genetic theory explains the accumulation of errors in the formation of new cells. However, the variety of these errors depend on lifestyle, environment, food habits, exposure to toxins, etc. and ought to lead to a diversity of manifestations in the aging process, yet we observe that aging is similar in presentation in all organisms.

Somehow, even small children can differentiate between a young person and an old person, demonstrating the uniform presentation of aging.

All people develop wrinkles as they age, eventually lose their reproductive ability, have gray hair, accumulate more fat, etc. There are processes that occur in every higher organism with the advancement of age, and these cannot be explained by random mutations.

The developmental-regulatory theory of aging explains this process from the point of view of regulatory processes that happen in every organism.

As we know, there are three major homeostatic systems (also called *homeostats*) in the living organism, namely energy, adaptation, and procreation. Gradual changes are necessary for growth and development to transform a fertilized egg into a fully grown organism capable of reproduction. These gradual changes are accomplished by the gradual increase in capacity of all three homeostatic systems, without which growth and development are impossible. The changes that lead to the acquisition of the ability to procreate are beneficial from the evolutionary point of view because they guarantee the survival of the species. However, the processes of continuous increase in the capacity of all three homeostats do not cease after the achievement of reproductive age—they continue past that point. And at some point, developmental changes start becoming detrimental, leading to stable disturbance of homeostasis (a disease) and eventually death.

From the evolutionary point of view, these changes guarantee the eventual loss of reproductive capacity, which is beneficial because with the advancement of age, the number of congenital birth defects increases, leading to unhealthy progeny.

The dying off of older animals guarantees that the food supply of a population remains adequate for the support of new, developing, and young reproducing organisms.

The similar changes that occur in all three homeostats simultaneously and synchronously led Dr. Dilman to believe that they originate from a single source. In his view, the only single organ in the body that regulates all three homeostats is the hypothalamus. He concluded that the organ responsible for the process of aging is the hypothalamus.

We cannot deny the importance of all these theories in an explanation of the phenomenon of aging, but the developmental-regulatory theory has a more comprehensive and uniform understanding of aging, at least at this point in time.

Chapter 9

The Law of Deviation of Homeostasis

The Law of Deviation of Homeostasis was postulated by Russian scientist, Dr. Vladimir Dilman, in the 1970s to integrate two seemingly mutually exclusive processes in the organism: the maintenance of homeostasis, and the process of growth and development.

We know that maintaining homeostasis, a steady state of the internal environment, is vitally important for the survival of the organism. At the same time, if something is stable, it is fixed, immovable, and unchanging. Growth and development is a process of continuous change, but a state of stability precludes change and therefore does not permit growth and development.

Thus, we have a paradox: If life is only possible under the condition that the internal environment remain stable, then growth and development are impossible without disturbance of this stability.

How do we develop from the fertilized cell into a fully grown organism capable of procreating, while maintaining the stability of the internal environment?

The process of development requires an increase of capacity of the system, which would be prohibited by homeostasis. Therefore, there must be some mechanism allowing change while maintaining a steady state.

The discovery of this mechanism was Dilman's fundamental contribution to science. He postulated that even though the steady state of the internal environment is maintained at any given moment, over time, the capacity of our main homeostat increases, allowing for growth. In effect, this process can be demonstrated in all three major homeostats—adaptation, energy, and reproduction. Homeostat being a self-organizing system that maintains certain quantities in state of homeostasis.

Let us go back to our bathroom and illustrate this mechanism using the bathroom tank as an example.

Imagine that our tank is slowly, but constantly, growing in size— the amount of water in the tank necessary to stop the influx of water slowly and gradually increases. At any given moment, water level is maintained by a negative feedback mechanism, but the system's capacity is increasing along with the growth of the volume of water. Looking at this phenomenon from the other point of view, the sensitivity of the tank to water decreases, meaning that a larger amount of water is needed to move the float upward in order to stop the influx. The same thing happens in the hormonal system. The hypothalamus very slowly becomes less and less sensitive to the negative feedback action of hormones. Dilman explains this change in sensitivity by changes in levels of neurotransmitters within the hypothalamus. It was proven that the hypothalamus of a younger animal is more sensitive to the action of peripheral hormones than the hypothalamus of an older animal. The gradual loss of hypothalamic sensitivity is why our development can occur while a steady state of the internal environment is being maintained.

We develop a larger body size with the passage of time. We utilize more energy, our sexual system gradually develops to allow procreation, and our ability to protect ourselves in times of adverse conditions increases. All this requires an increased potency in all three major homeostats (energy, procreation, and adaptation). This gradual shift requires years and occurs slowly, all the while maintaining a stable state of the internal environment.

When growth of the body stops, this gradual increase in capacity of the homeostats does not stop but continues at the same pace. While it was necessary for the growth and development of the body for achieving a reproductive state, it becomes the main factor leading to the disruption of all homeostats after the growth process comes to an end.

Since this shift occurs in all homeostats simultaneously, there must be one organ in the body that controls all of them simultaneously. The only organ that controls all of them is the hypothalamus. It is here that this gradual change must originate.

The proof of this phenomenon came from the scientific experiments confirming the fact that the hypothalamus gradually becomes less and less sensitive to the action of hormones. In order to maintain the negative feedback mechanisms, it requires higher and higher levels of hormones to stop the hypothalamic stimulation of the glands.

One experiment was to compare the sensitivity of the adrenal system to the level of the hormone cortisol. In order to do this, scientists use the dexamethasone suppression test. Dexamethasone is a derivative of cortisol and similarly acts on the hypothalamo-pituitary-adrenal system. However, cortisol and dexamethasone require different tests to measure their levels. The cortisol level declines after injection of dexamethasone, which acts on the hypothalamus like cortisol but does not interfere with the cortisol test.

Dexamethasone was found to suppress cortisol levels by 51% in 2-month-old rats, but the suppression decreased to 11% in 8-month-old rats. Similar results were observed in humans. Dexamethasone suppressed the concentration of cortisol by 47% in 30-year-olds, but the suppression decreased to 33% in 50-year-olds.

This study shows that the hypothalamus of older animals is much less sensitive to the action of dexamethasone—and therefore cortisol—than that of younger ones.

The idea that changes in the hypothalamus are what drives development presents another question.

What exactly happens in the hypothalamus that increases the capacity of the main homeostat? What causes this loss of sensitivity?

Here we need to reiterate that the hypothalamus is part of the nervous system and consists of nerve cells that lose the ability to divide with aging.

This is not true of the pituitary, which is a gland and has the capacity to increase both the volume and number of its cells, thus allowing for increased capacity while preserving precise regulation by the hypothalamus.

There are also certain changes that occur in the hypothalamus with aging.

Each nerve cell is like a microscopic endocrine gland producing hormone-like substances, called neurotransmitters. Neurotransmitters transfer specific signals from one nerve cell to another. Strictly speaking, neurons do not form a continuous electrical circuit. They connect to each other by way of synapses, which are microscopic gaps between the cells. To transmit a signal, a neuron releases a neurotransmitter into the synapse. The receiving neuron has receptors that respond to neurotransmitters. This chemical signal generates an electrical impulse inside a neuron so it can further transmit the signal.

There are numerous neurotransmitters that either stimulate or inhibit neuronal activity. There are also several factors that may change the sensitivity of the regulator.

The first of these factors is a decrease in the number of receptors, decreasing the number of molecules of a neurotransmitter that can connect to a receptor, leading to decreased sensitivity. It is a rule that an increase in the concentration of any hormone, including neurotransmitters, results in a decrease in the number of receptors to protect a cell from excess effect.

The second factor is related to the maturation and aging of neurons. As they age, they accumulate cholesterol in their plasma membranes, resulting in a decreased ability of receptors to respond to neurotransmitters.

The third factor is a decrease of available neurotransmitters, which occurs with age.

Each of these factors makes the hypothalamus less sensitive to hormones, requiring an increase of their concentration to execute negative feedback.

Thus, the requirement of a stable internal environment at any given moment is coupled with a gradual increase in the capacity of the system, allowing for growth and development.

The Law of Deviation of Homeostasis not only explains how growth can be achieved without violation of homeostasis, but it also explains the phenomenon of aging from the point of view of regulation of processes in the body.

The main point of Dilman's theory of aging is that aging occurs simultaneously in all three major functions of life, three homeostats. As we age, our ability to procreate diminishes. Women go into menopause. Men's sexual drive and ability gradually diminishes and ceases at some point in life. Changes in energy exchange lead to the accumulation of fat and the development of pre-diabetes, diabetes, and atherosclerosis. We have a harder time adjusting to adverse conditions.

These changes occur in different organs and different homeostats simultaneously. The only organ in the body where all three systems are regulated is the hypothalamus. It is easy to conclude, therefore, that the only organ in the body that can influence all three homeostats at once is the hypothalamus. Continuous changes in the hypothalamus cause an organism's initial growth and development—and its subsequent aging and decline.

Chapter 10

Testosterone

AB, at the age of 48, was not the man he used to be. He started to feel that his well-being was declining. All his adult life, he had gone to a gym daily to work out, but lately, it took effort to make himself go exercise. His muscles, especially around the shoulders, started to thin, and he became generally weaker. Even though he could no longer lift as heavy weights, his muscles and joints became more and more achy after a workout.

He had been used to being very active but now preferred to spend time sitting on the couch, watching TV. Even going to a party took effort. He became more nervous and irritable, and his wife complained of him being a grumpy old man. Hair disappeared from his calves, and he looked pale. He started to gain some fat on his breasts and lower abdomen. What worried him most is that his sexual desire had almost disappeared, and he was not able to perform in bed like he used to, even though he could maintain an erection. He used to wake up with an erection, but for the last several years, this had become rarer and rarer.

He felt depressed, over-the-hill, that he had passed his peak.

AB was suffering from low testosterone.

What makes a man different from a woman?

He has testicles and a penis and does not have a vagina and ovaries.

A man has wider shoulders and smaller hips. He has bigger and stronger muscles, less fatty tissue, and more red blood cells. He has a beard and more body hair. He is more prone to risky behavior and naturally strives to dominate. He is always looking for an opportunity to mate with a female or get into a fight or a competition with another male. He loves a challenge. His hair recedes on his temples and crown with age. His bones are thicker, and his breasts are smaller. His voice is deeper.

All these features are results of actions of the male hormone, testosterone, which is produced mostly in the testicles but also in small amounts in adrenal glands. Females also produce some testosterone in their ovaries and adrenal glands, but about ten times less.

Testosterone was first isolated by Ernst Laqueur and his group. In 1935, they used 100 kg (220 pounds) of bull testicles to isolate 10 milligrams of a potent new androgen and named it testosterone. In the same year, Adolf Butenandt and Leopold Ruzicka synthesized testosterone independently of each other and using different pathways.

Ruzicka used a method in which the precursor of testosterone was methyltestosterone, the first orally effective testosterone preparation, which was subsequently abandoned due to its toxicity to the liver.

Testosterone is the primary male sex hormone and an anabolic steroid.

As a male hormone, it induces the development and maintenance of male qualities. This includes the development of male sex organs before birth as well as secondary sex characteristics, such as the male hair patterns of the beard, chest, and extremities, male pattern balding, larger chin and brow, etc.

Testosterone is anabolic in that it increases the production of protein in cells that have testosterone receptors, causing them to grow. This is why males have larger and stronger muscles than females. It promotes bone growth and increases bone density. It stimulates bone maturation. Boys whose puberty starts late are taller because they have more time to grow than those with early-onset puberty.

Testosterone levels in boys rise right after birth and remain high for several months, diminishing to almost undetectable by 4 to 6 months. After that, they remain very low, rising very slowly until puberty.

Right before puberty, testosterone levels rapidly rise in both boys and girls. The increase in testosterone levels causes them to have oily skin and hair and develop acne.

At the same time, pubic and armpit hair start to appear, and they acquire adult-type body odor.

As puberty advances, testicles mature and the production of sperms begins. Penis and clitoris increase in size. Libido increases, and erection of penis or engorgement of clitoris occur more often. Facial structure in boys changes, with the growth of the jaw, brow, chin, and nose. Bones mature and growth zones calcify, and rapid growth slows down and eventually stops.

After puberty, testosterone levels fluctuate depending on the situation. For example, testosterone levels rise during hard physical exercise. When a male is winning in a competition with a challenging counterpart, he has a very steep rise in testosterone, but if he is losing, testosterone levels drop.

Marriage and fatherhood decrease testosterone levels.

Interestingly enough, males are sensitive to the menstrual cycle of females, and their testosterone rises when their partner is ovulating. Testosterone levels start diminishing after the age of 30.

In females, menopause develops rather abruptly, along with symptoms of rapid hormone loss, such as the absence of menstruation, hot flashes, and night sweats, among others.

In males, however, the process is gradual, with a slow decline of testosterone levels at a rate of 1 to 2% a year. It takes many years of decline for symptoms to become bothersome. An analogy of the proverbial frog comes to mind. When it was placed in a pot of water with the temperature rising slowly, the frog would not know when it was boiled.

This is why the male counterpart of menopause, andropause, did not receive appropriate attention from the medical community until very recently.

As the male ages, his testosterone slowly declines, resulting in the loss of the typical male characteristics. A man starts to accumulate fat, his muscles become thinner and weaker, especially in the shoulders, his red blood cells diminish in number, and he looks paler. He becomes inactive, lazy, and indecisive. His desire and ability for mating wanes. He becomes anxious, nervous, and grumpy.

Symptoms of low testosterone are very similar to symptoms of metabolic syndrome (increase in abdominal girth, high LDL cholesterol, high blood pressure, elevated sugar levels), which is a condition associated with increased mortality. Testosterone has been proven to reverse metabolic syndrome, support the heart and sexual functions, lower blood pressure, improve cholesterol, and help with sugar and weight control. It has antidepressant qualities, improves sleep, and increases muscle strength and the desire to exercise.

Recently, a worrisome phenomenon has been discovered. Scientists compared mean levels of testosterone in men of age-matched groups in 1987-1989, 1995-1997, and 2002-2004. In all age-matched groups, testosterone declined at a speed of 1.2%. This was *in addition* to the age-related decline of 1 to 2% per year.

This study showed that any man today has roughly 50% lower testosterone than an equal-age man from 40 years ago. The same pattern is happening with sperm counts.

As a main "male hormone," testosterone is a very important hormone for men, but it also is very important for women, even though testosterone levels in women is 1/7 to 1/10 that of a man. Firstly, the female hormone estradiol is made from testosterone.

Testosterone modulates the physiology of vaginal tissues. It is essential in maintaining muscles and bones in females too. It slows the thinning of the skin.

It contributes a great deal to female sexual arousal and libido. It has antidepressant and anti-anxiety effects in females, just like in males.

A recent study shows that testosterone plays an important role in the prenatal (prior to birth) development of females. Low testosterone levels of the mother lead to the development of endometriosis, a painful condition when the uterine lining grows outside of the uterus. High testosterone is implicated in the development of polycystic ovarian syndrome, a disease where females develop cysts in the ovaries and produce too much testosterone.

Testosterone receptors are present in large numbers in the brain, and the key cognitive functions affected by testosterone in humans are attention, memory, and spatial ability. There is some evidence that low testosterone levels are a risk factor for development of cognitive decline and dementia.

Chapter 11

Estrogen

C S, a mother of 2 and a busy businesswoman, came to her doctor with complaints of being tired. This fatigue was not the kind that appears after an exhausting day at work and that disappears after a good sleep. It seemed to affect her 24 hours a day. She also started to have hot flashes and problems sleeping, awakening from night sweats. She used to have regular periods that came like clockwork every 28 days, but now she occasionally missed a period or had it too early, and this was becoming more and more frequent. Recently, she did not have a period for three months. Her breasts began to droop, but occasionally they would become heavy and tender, and she started to have pain during sex with her husband due to the dryness of her vagina. She also started to have dry eyes, but it was not bothersome enough to seek the consultation of an eye doctor. Her hair started to thin, and hair loss increased, especially on top of her head. Her skin started to thin, and small wrinkles started to appear on her upper lip.

She felt somewhat depressed and noticed a lack of memory and concentration at work. She became very irritable and tearful.

CS was suffering from estrogen imbalance related to menopause.

Just as there is a male hormone, testosterone, there is a female counterpart, estrogen.

Estrogen is found in three major forms.

1. Estrone (ES-tr-one), the main estrogen after menopause

2. Estradiol (es-tra-Di-ol), the most active estrogen, the one that is responsible for most of the feminizing effects.

3. Estriol (ES-tri-ol), the main estrogen in premenopausal women. This one is a very weak estrogen. It could be thought of as anti-estrogen because it occupies estrogen receptors but is eight times weaker than estradiol. Estriol is the estrogen that maintains skin and mucosal membranes such as vaginal mucosa and others.

The discovery of female hormones is dated to 1929, when two scientists, Edward Doisy and Alfred Butenandt, independently—and almost simultaneously—purified and crystalized estrone. Doisy later discovered estriol and estradiol.

Estradiol is the predominant sex hormone in females but is also present in males, though in much smaller amounts. It is produced from the male hormone testosterone, mostly in the ovaries and in small amounts in the adrenal glands, testicles, and fat tissue.

In contrast to testosterone, estradiol promotes the development of female sex characteristics. It promotes typical female fat deposits in breasts and hips rather than in the abdomen, which is typical for males. It plays a vital role in the growth and development of female sexual organs and their inner lining and the development of breasts and nipples. It causes the hair to grow in a typical female pattern, mostly in the pubic and armpit areas. It makes female joints more flexible. It takes part in triggering ovulation and maintaining pregnancy.

Estradiol is the hormone that promotes the growth of the endometrium, the inner lining of the uterus, to replace the old one that was rejected during the last menstruation.

It has an antidepressant and energizing effect on the female brain. The lack of estradiol is associated with a characteristic 24-hour-a-day fatigue, mental fog, and memory lapses.

Estradiol levels are not stable but regularly fluctuate with the progression of the menstrual cycle.

All these effects are diminished during menopause, when production of estradiol falls.

Estradiol promotes the deposition of calcium into bones in females and males, which is why individuals with low estradiol during the growth period grow taller. Their bones have more time to grow before they are totally calcified. When estradiol levels decrease during menopause, calcium starts to leave bone tissue, and women gradually develop osteoporosis—their bones become more fragile.

Estradiol is a moisturizing hormone; it causes retention of water.

Without it (when estradiol production ceases during and after menopause), the vaginal lining becomes dry, breasts droop, and eyes lose their sparkle due to lack of tears. In contrast, just before the menstrual period, when there are high levels of estradiol, breasts, fingers, and legs may swell.

Estradiol is an important factor in support of hair, and women lacking estradiol often have thinning hair on the top of their heads, but not on the temples and crowns like males.

Estradiol has a profound effect on the skin. Aside from its moisturizing effects, estradiol supports the integrity of collagen fibers that constitute the structural matrix of the skin. After the beginning of menopause, skin becomes progressively thinner and wrinkle formation increases. One of the symptoms of menopause is the appearance of thin vertical wrinkles of the upper lip of some women, that many people mistakenly think is caused by smoking.

Exposure to estradiol protects skin from accelerated aging, increasing skin elasticity, thickness, and strength.

Estradiol also causes softening and dissolution of atherosclerotic plaques in the blood vessels, which makes the hormone protective, from the point of view of the heart. However, it may increase the frequency of heart attacks in women who start taking estradiol at an age older than 65, when plaques are already formed, and thinning may trigger the bursting of the plaque and result in a heart attack.

Estradiol has a profound effect on the brain, acting not only as a hormone but also as a neurotransmitter involved in learning and memory, acting almost instantly. Estradiol was shown to improve memory and cognitive function in older women with mild symptoms of dementia and Alzheimer's disease. Healthy estradiol levels are associated with feelings of well-being and good mood. Sudden drops of estradiol, as well as sustained long-term low levels, are associated with symptoms of depression.

Contrary to popular belief, it is not testosterone but estradiol that creates and increases sex drive in females as well as in males. So why does testosterone, more than estradiol, increase sex drive?

This peculiarity can be explained by a high concentration of aromatase (the enzyme that converts testosterone into estradiol) in the brain area responsible for libido. This conversion occurs at a very high rate, and more estradiol is created from testosterone there than is available from the general circulation. This is why an increase in testosterone concentration in the blood leads to an exponential increase of estradiol around the hypothalamus.

Determination of masculinization in the human brain is not completely understood, but an interesting mechanism of this process was discovered in mice.

Before birth, female mouse fetuses produce a large amount of a special protein called alpha-fetoprotein. This protein prevents estradiol from reaching the brain of female fetuses but not male ones. When estradiol reaches the brain of the male fetuses, it produces a masculinizing effect on their brains.

Chapter 12

Progesterone

After her 45th birthday, Lisa still had regular menstrual periods, but something changed in her life. Occasionally, 2 to 3 days before her period started, she became very irritable, tearful, impatient, and nervous. She quarreled with no apparent reason with her husband and often cried during their arguments. Her breasts became very tender and heavy, and rings were tight on her fingers. A good sleeper, she could not fall asleep during these days, and even if she would, she would wake up several times in the middle of the night. She started to bleed very heavily and with clots. Her periods became longer and lasted for seven days, when usually her period lasted only 4 or 5, and she did not bleed that much. She started to gain weight but mostly in her lower belly and thighs.

Two or three days after her period started, she would become her usual self again.

Her doctor reassured her that it was just PMS (premenstrual syndrome), which was normal at her age.

At first, she had it rather rarely, but gradually it became more and more frequent, and now she has it almost every menstrual cycle.

Explanation: Her ovaries started to misfire occasionally, and some cycles were proceeding without ovulation. During these anovulatory cycles, she did not make enough progesterone, and that explained her symptoms.

Progesterone was first isolated by W.M. Allen and G.W. Corner in 1929. Several groups of investigators were working on its discovery between 1928 and 1934, but again it was Adolf Butenandt who was first to describe the structural formula of progesterone, in 1934.

Progesterone used to be thought of as a pregnancy hormone because its production is closely related to ovulation and pregnancy. But it is more than a maternity hormone. It plays an important role in females and males. In males, it is produced in the adrenal glands and the testicles. Progesterone levels in men are the same as in post-menopausal women.

Progesterone occupies a central position in the steroidogenic cascade. Most of the steroid hormones can be, and are, made of progesterone, such as cortisol, aldosterone, and even testosterone and estrogens. Altogether, there are around 40 different steroid hormones that are produced in different stages of the process of steroid synthesis.

Progesterone is produced directly from pregnenolone, the "mother" hormone, from which all steroid hormones are made. Progesterone is just one step away from pregnenolone and two steps away from cholesterol.

Like most animals, women produce eggs. When an egg is about ready to be released, a little bubble (follicle) forms around it and continues to grow until it bursts and releases an egg to be fertilized.

When a follicle bursts, a scar forms in its place that has a characteristically yellow color and is called the corpus luteum ("yellow body" in Latin), which is biologically active and produces a large amount of progesterone. Progesterone makes the endometrium, the inner lining of the uterus, soft, bulky (ripe), and hospitable to the fertilized egg. This allows an egg to implant easily into the endometrium and start dividing.

If an egg is not fertilized, the corpus luteum disappears, the production of progesterone stops, and the endometrium is rejected, causing menstruation to start. If conception occurs, the corpus luteum continues to function throughout the first trimester of pregnancy and then undergoes involution—it disappears. In the second and third trimesters, a large amount of progesterone is produced in the placenta, which is formed by the time the corpus luteum disappears. Progesterone keeps the cervix of the uterus closed, which prevents miscarriage. It is the action of high levels of progesterone that make the characteristic changes in the appearance of pregnant women, which are easily recognizable, like darkening of nipples and body folds (armpits and perineum) and increased size of nose and chin.

Progesterone belongs to a triad of hormones called neurosteroids.

They are produced not only in the ovaries and adrenal glands but also synthesized in the brain and profoundly affect brain function, acting as neurotransmitters.

It has been demonstrated that progesterone in the nervous system works similarly to well-known medications such as Valium and Xanax, attaching to GABA receptors in the brain, improving sleep and relieving irritability, nervousness, and anxiety. Indeed, the lack of progesterone results in the opposite effects.

In addition, progesterone has been proven to help with pain due to acute back pain attacks, and diabetic and other neuropathies by restoring and rebuilding of myelin cover of nerve fibers. By the same action, progesterone may slow the progression of Alzheimer's disease and other nervous system ailments.

It has been theorized that a sudden drop in progesterone levels after childbirth takes part in the development of post-partum depression because progesterone has anti-depressive qualities. Another important role of progesterone in men and women is that it inhibits the overreaction of immune cells, and this explains why most autoimmune disorders such as lupus and rheumatoid arthritis are less severe during pregnancy when progesterone levels are high.

Progesterone can attach to cortisol receptors and occupy them and thus can have mild anti-cortisol action. Progesterone improves breathing function by inducing mild hyperventilation and is used occasionally to treat COPD.

Progesterone levels in men are similar to levels in postmenopausal women, which proves the importance of progesterone in men.

In men, progesterone activates spermatozoids and makes them capable of penetrating into the female's egg.

Signs of progesterone deficiency in men include a combination of early balding and increased body hair, especially on the back. Those are signs of a high level of testosterone metabolite DHT (dihydrotestosterone), the most potent androgen in the body, which is toxic to hair follicles of the scalp but promotes the growth of body hair. Progesterone partially blocks the conversion of testosterone into DHT, thus protecting the follicles from dying. DHT, as the most potent androgen, is responsible for body hair growth, and this explains a very hairy back and shoulders in progesterone-deficient males.

As a precursor hormone, progesterone acts as a building material for most steroid hormones, particularly cortisol, a stress and defense hormone. As a result, chronic stress leads to decreased levels of progesterone due to increased conversion into cortisol. This drop in progesterone levels can contribute to an occasional inability to conceive or maintain pregnancy during stressful times.

Chapter 13

Regulation of Reproductive Function

Reproduction, like all other homeostats, undergoes deep changes throughout the process of development, maturation, and decline of an organism.

Mammals, like most complex organisms, are unable to reproduce at birth.

Their hypothalamus is extremely sensitive to negative feedback, and the lowest levels of sex hormones are able to exercise inhibition of the production of stimulating hormones, gonadotropins.

As an animal matures, the hypothalamus becomes less and less sensitive to the action of sex hormones, and higher levels are required in order to stop stimulation of their production.

In an experiment, it took only about 0.5 micrograms of the sex hormone estradiol to slow down stimulation by half in a 1-month-old rat. It took four times more estradiol to achieve the same effect in an adult animal.

But if the sensitivity of the hypothalamus gradually declines, more and more sex hormones will be needed to suppress the production of stimulating hormones. The hypothalamus gradually escapes from inhibition, and at some point, the increased production of sex hormones will cause the development of sexual characteristics. After a while, it will bring initiation of reproductive function.

Thus, the mechanism of sexual development is based on the phenomenon of a gradual decline of hypothalamic sensitivity to the suppressive action of sex hormones. This is the only way that allows an increase in the power of the system while maintaining a mechanism of self-regulation.

But with the increasing power of the system due to a decrease of hypothalamic sensitivity, peripheral hormones become unable to suppress stimulation. As a result, stimulating hormones, gonadotropins, will be produced in larger and larger quantities, making glands produce more and more hormones.

In males, sexual development is straightforward. After achieving sexual maturation, the ever-decreasing hypothalamic sensitivity leads to an increase in the production of gonadotropins and the male hormone testosterone. At a certain point, testicles would be unable to produce more testosterone in response to increased levels of stimulating hormones. After working in a regime of maximal capacity for a while, testicles become worn out and are able to produce less and less testosterone. Its level gradually declines, leading to testosterone deficiency and loss of capacity to reproduce.

We may ask why males retain reproductive ability so much longer than females. We see some men still having children at the age of 60— sometimes even later.

The answer is that having children past the period of top performance is a purely human phenomenon. In the animal kingdom, males subjected to gradual loss of testosterone develop typical symptoms of hypogonadism. They become weaker, slower, less assertive, their ability to procure food diminishes, and they cannot compete with younger contenders for the privilege of mating. They never reach the state of old age, and die when falling prey to predators, disease, or male competitors.

There is a peculiarity, though, in the development of sexual and reproductive functions in females.

In contrast with males, females not only have a tonic (meaning continuous or steady) mechanism in the hypothalamus that works just like in males, but they also have a cyclical mechanism which is responsible for menstrual cycles and production of eggs.

When the tonic mechanism becomes developed enough, increasing levels of sex hormones cause the development of secondary sexual characteristics such as pubic and armpit hair, breast, and general female body structure. After these changes are accomplished, the continuously rising level of the sex hormone estradiol turns on the function of the cyclical center in the hypothalamus. This is achieved by the mechanism of positive (stimulating) feedback, the opposite of negative feedback.

This means that a certain level of estradiol needs to be achieved in order to start activity of the cyclic center.

This cyclic mechanism is responsible for the fluctuations of female hormones that lead to ovulation and pregnancy.

The cyclic center is regulated by the same mechanism as other hormones, namely hypothalamus-pituitary-ovary. It is also subject to the ever-decreasing sensitivity of the hypothalamus to the action of sex hormones.

Let us examine how an increase in production of sex hormones during the whole reproductive period, roughly 30 years, allows overcoming these hypothalamic changes.

Despite achievement of reproductive age, hypothalamic sensitivity in 3-month-old rats continues to decline. This fact was confirmed by an experiment that demonstrated that the dose of sex hormones necessary to suppress the tonic center increases with the increasing age of the animal. In other words, the decline in sensitivity of the hypothalamus after turning on reproductive function does not halt but continues to progress.

At the same time, the cyclic center becomes less and less sensitive, and it requires more and more sex hormones to trigger ovulation. For about 30 years, this is compensated by the increase in the ability of the ovaries to produce more and more sex hormones. But at some point, even these high levels of hormones are unable to start the activity of the cyclical center, and ovulation does not occur. The cessation of ovulation marks the onset of menopause.

This mechanism can explain how a gradual decrease of hypothalamic sensitivity to the action of peripheral hormones initially ensures the age-related switching on, and then the age-related switching-off, of reproductive function.

It was confirmed by an experiment conducted by the Japanese scientist Kushima who spayed female rats of two age groups, young and old, and then transplanted the ovaries of the young rats into the old ones. If the ability to ovulate depended on the age of the ovaries, this operation would restore old rats' reproductive activity. That did not happen. Old rats did not restart their cycles.

However, when the ovaries of old rats were transplanted into young animals, they started to function. This experiment confirmed that it is the aging of the hypothalamus and not the ovaries that induce the development of menopause.

The switching off of reproductive function is biologically beneficial for the following reasons.

It regulates the number of organisms in the population, contributing to maintaining an optimum quantity for a given living space.

It reduces the possibility of birth defects, which are more common with the advancing age of a mother.

It regulates the rate of succession of generations, which increases the rate of exchange of genetic material to maximize the chance to get beneficial combinations of genes.

Chapter 14

Thyroid Hormone

Several months ago, Bertha started to feel cold most of the time, even when everybody else in the room was comfortable. She noticed that she felt very tired, especially when she woke up. It was hard to get out of bed in the morning. As she started to move around doing her morning routine, her fatigue felt better, and she regained some energy. Throughout the day, she felt somewhat better when moving around, but after several minutes without moving, like while driving or watching TV, she felt increasing fatigue and the desire to sleep or just lay down.

She started to gain weight even though her diet did not change. She tried to eat less but to no avail—she kept gaining. She became somewhat constipated and did not have a bowel movement every day like she used to have. Her hair started to fall out, and her periods became irregular. Her thought processes also became slow, and work productivity dropped. Her doctor mentioned that her pulse got slower, and her temperature never went above 98.0. She developed bags under her eyes, and her eyebrows started to thin from the outside.

She became depressed and looked a bit swollen.

Bertha was experiencing typical symptoms of low thyroid hormone.

Thyroid hormone, thyroxine (T4), was first isolated in 1915 by an American chemist, Edward Kendall.

It is produced in the thyroid gland, located in the lower part of the throat. It is regulated by a pituitary hormone called thyroid stimulating hormone (TSH or thyrotropin) which, in its turn, is controlled by thyrotropin releasing factor from the hypothalamus. The normal function of thyroid hormones is very much dependent on iodine intake. Too much or too little iodine results in thyroid abnormalities.

The thyroid hormone that is released into blood consists of a small molecule, thyronine, made from the same amino acid (tyrosine) as the adrenal hormones epinephrine, norepinephrine, and the neurotransmitter of pleasure, dopamine. Four atoms of iodine are attached to thyronine, making it into 4-iodothyronine. This is why doctors usually call this hormone "T4".

T4 can be considered a pro-hormone. It is stored inside the thyroid gland and released into the bloodstream. It is converted to an active form in the cells by removing 1 of its iodine atoms, turning it into T3, 3-iodothyronine, which is four times more active than T4. This reaction requires selenium, an important microelement. The thyroid also releases some T3 into the bloodstream—but only a tiny amount.

Thyroid hormones are very poorly soluble in water, with only 0.03% of T4 and 0.3% of T3 circulating in the blood in biologically active form. Most T4 and T3 circulate in the blood while attached to transport proteins, making them inactive.

Thyroid hormone—in particular, T3—increases the speed of chemical reactions in the body (basic metabolic rate) by increasing the rate of utilization of oxygen, which results in faster burning of foodstuffs and a rise in body temperature.

The faster chemical reactions run, the higher the temperature. The action of thyroid hormone can be compared to airflow in a furnace.

Thyroid hormone

1. *increases cardiac output, heart rate, and breathing,*
1. *increases the effects of catecholamine hormones—epinephrine and norepinephrine,*
1. *is essential for brain development,*
1. *thickens the endometrium in females,*
1. *increases the catabolism of proteins and carbohydrates,*
1. *affects protein synthesis and long bone growth,*
1. *is involved in development of hair and skin, such as fur molting in mammals and skin shedding in reptiles,*
1. *takes part in steroid hormone production and breakdown.*

Thus, the main function of the thyroid gland is to increase the speed with which your body operates.

With too little thyroid hormone, everything in the body is slow: burning calories, movements, thoughts, heart rate, etc. Conversely, with too much of this hormone, everything is too fast.

Usually, people who have too little thyroid hormone are always cold. Their heart rate is unusually slow, and their temperature is low. They are unable to lose weight even when on a diet because they burn foodstuffs very slowly. Their movements are slow, and they are constipated because their intestines move too slowly too. They always feel tired, but the worst fatigue is upon awakening. This morning fatigue gets better when they start moving, when increased circulation brings more thyroid hormone to their cells. But as soon as they stop moving, fatigue returns, as when sitting or lying down. In severe cases, they accumulate jelly-like substance everywhere in the body, and this extreme degree of thyroid deficiency, which is life-threatening, is called myxedema. Due to slow thinking, their mental abilities decline. More often than not, they are depressed.

The other symptoms are thinning of the outer parts of the eyebrows, slow reflexes, and yellowing of the soles. Thyroid hormone helps to convert carotene, an orange pigment found in abundance in carrots and turmeric, into vitamin A. Too much carotene colors the soles of the feet yellowish orange.

The thyroid hormone is very important for hair. People whose thyroid hormone is too low (or too high) complain of thinning or falling out hair.

Symptoms of excessive thyroid hormone have the opposite set of symptoms: always feeling hot, racing thoughts, fast heart rate, increased temperature, fast movements, shaking muscles, nervousness, loose bowel movements, inability to sleep, weight loss, and bulging eyes.

Thyroid hormones are essential for the mental development of children. Low thyroid levels in the womb result in a syndrome of congenital hypothyroidism (formerly called cretinism) with severe mental retardation, a large swollen tongue that sometimes cannot fit inside the mouth and sticks out, flat feet, increased flexibility of joints, and other face and bony abnormalities.

Thyroid abnormalities are a frequent cause of menstrual irregularities in women.

With age, the production of thyroid hormone and conversion of T4 to T3 declines, which contributes to loss of energy, thinning hair, depression, mental decline, and increased weight, blood sugar, and triglycerides. These age-related changes are called sub-clinical hypothyroidism because, despite typical symptoms, thyroid hormones and TSH remain within reference ranges.

Usually, doctors measure only thyroid stimulating hormone as an indicator of thyroid health. But checking levels of free/unbound T4 and T3 and an inactive form of T3, reverse T3, is necessary to assess thyroid function.

The best way to check your thyroid activity at home is to check your temperature upon waking. If it is low, your thyroid is most likely underactive.

Chapter 15

Insulin and Glucagon

Insulin is considered to be the main anabolic hormone in the body, which means that it induces the creation of larger, more complicated molecules from smaller ones. It also acts as a very important part of the energy homeostat.

It is a peptide hormone produced in beta cells in the pancreas and is released in response to an increase in sugar levels in the bloodstream.

Insulin drives molecules of glucose from the bloodstream into cells of the liver, muscles, and fatty tissue.

Upon entering the muscle cells, glucose is either burned for energy or is converted into the animal starch, glycogen, for later use. In the fatty tissue, it is converted into triglycerides (neutral fats) and stored. In the case of the liver, it can be converted into either.

Insulin rapidly activates protein synthesis and increases the number of ribosomes, the protein-creating organelles inside the cell.

Insulin is a very greedy hormone. Once sugar is converted to fat, it impedes the release of fat from fatty tissue into blood, acting toward energy sources like a greedy and stingy person who is trying to endlessly acquire more money and avoid parting with it.

When the concentration of sugars and fatty acids in the bloodstream increases, insulin is rapidly released into the blood by beta cells and activates the transport of sugars and fatty acids into cells.

Insulin acts in opposition to growth hormone, which releases fatty acids in response to declining sugar levels.

If an auto-immune process destroys beta cells, production of insulin is impaired, and glucose cannot move from the bloodstream into the cells, thus causing blood sugar levels to rise. This condition is called diabetes mellitus type 1 (previously called "juvenile" because it usually develops at a young age). This type of diabetes is very different from type 2 diabetes, which is caused by an excess amount of fat in the body, leading to more glucose in the blood than the body can use for energy. An increased amount of insulin is necessary to remove extra sugar from the bloodstream, further increasing the size of the fat cells. The membranes of fat cells expand, the receptors become sparse, and cells stop responding to insulin signaling. This causes further elevation of insulin levels in an attempt to remove glucose.

At a certain point, even an elevated concentration of insulin is not enough to remove most of the sugar from the blood. A condition called insulin resistance develops, leading to type 2 diabetes.

Glucagon is a hormone that acts opposite to insulin. Glucagon is produced by alpha cells in the pancreas, and it causes the increased production and release of sugar from the liver into the bloodstream. This happens in response to the release of epinephrine and norepinephrine during the early stages of stress, and in cases when blood glucose levels fall dangerously low.

Chapter 16

Growth Hormone (GH)

Most of us have seen pictures of the tallest man who ever lived, Robert Wadlow, who was 8 feet, 11.1 inches tall as measured on June 27, 1940—less than one inch from 9 feet tall. Charles S. Stratton (born February 4, 1838), nicknamed General Tom Thumb, is the most famous short man. His height was 3 feet, 2 inches.

These men were both affected by disorders of growth hormone production from childhood. The first had too much and the second too little. These are extremes, caused by diseases of the pituitary gland resulting in abnormalities of growth hormone production and metabolism. However, people differ in body height from very short to very tall depending on the amount of growth hormone produced in their bodies and the time until bones are calcified and stop growing, which happens at the end of puberty.

At first, growth hormone was thought of as a hormone that promotes the linear growth of the body. Later, when the action of growth hormone was studied in more detail, it was determined that its function is much more fundamental than just regulating height.

It was discovered and isolated by Choh Hao Li in 1956. Growth hormone was determined to be species-specific, which is why growth hormones from cows or pigs did not work in humans. It was not until 1958 that the human growth hormone was isolated from human cadavers' pituitary glands. The chemical structure of the human growth hormone was identified in 1972.

Growth hormone is produced and stored in pituitary gland. Apparently, nature cared so much about this hormone that it did not delegate its production to a peripheral gland but made it a responsibility of the pituitary itself. The release of GH is regulated by hypothalamic GHRH (growth hormone releasing hormone).

Unlike steroid hormones, which are fat-soluble and easily penetrate cell membranes, growth hormone is a protein and is not fat-soluble. It cannot travel inside the cell and acts by interacting with specific growth hormone receptors on the surface of cells.

The daily production of growth hormone is about 330 micrograms, which is released mostly at night during sleep. This is why children are motivated to go to sleep early and told that they grow when they sleep.

Growth hormone has two major functions.

The first function is accomplished by growth hormone itself. GH is released into the bloodstream mostly at night and exists there only for 10 to 20 minutes. The release of GH is triggered by a drop in blood glucose level that occurs due to the nightly fast when we are asleep and unable to eat.

GH causes the release of fatty acids from fatty tissues into the bloodstream to feed cells at the time when glucose is in short supply. Fatty acids can easily penetrate inside the cell through membranes because cell membranes are made of fatty acids and cholesterol, and fat dissolves in fat. It only takes 4 to 6 minutes for fatty acids to be incorporated inside the cells. Sugar, in contrast, is water-soluble and cannot go directly through the cell membrane. It requires insulin to be transported into a cell, but when the level of sugar is low, the level of insulin is also low. During the night, sugar needs to be reserved for nervous tissue, which utilizes glucose as its main source of energy.

The other function of growth hormone is to stimulate the liver to produce insulin-like growth factor 1 or IGF-1.

IGF-1 is produced mostly by the liver throughout life. The highest levels of IGF-1 are detected during the growth spurt of puberty, and the lowest are in infancy and old age.

The role of IGF-1 is to stimulate growth, cell reproduction, and cell regeneration, and to lower the rate of programmed cell suicide (apoptosis) in humans and other animals. It sends the signal to cells that sufficient nutrients are available for cells to grow and divide.

IGF-1 has a growth-promoting effect on almost every cell in the body but especially skeletal muscles, cartilage, bone, liver, kidney, nerve tissue, skin, blood cell lines, and lung cells.

After age 25, production of GH starts to diminish, and by age 30, most everyone has a mild degree of GH deficiency. This decline continues throughout the rest of life. The lack of GH later in life is responsible for the shrinking of the tissues. We all know that at an older age we become shorter, and our muscles and skin become thinner.

In a person with a growth hormone deficiency, we notice thin skin with fine wrinkles, droopy eyelids, sagging cheeks, muscle wasting around shoulders and buttocks. Everything in the body is starting to hang because cells become smaller.

To check for growth hormone deficiency, anyone can pinch and hold the skin of the back of the hand and then release the pinch. If the fold stays longer than 4 seconds, a person is GH deficient.

This is why, to slow down shrinking, sagging, and hanging skin and to burn more fat, we need to stop eating 3 to 4 hours before bedtime to achieve the nightly drop in blood sugar leading to the release of growth hormone. This releases fats out of fatty tissue and raises the level of IGF-1 to promote maintenance of cells. However, even with our best efforts, the release of growth hormone at night diminishes with age.

Like most hormones, growth hormone has a pronounced effect on the nervous system. It stimulates the parasympathetic system, the calming half of the autonomic nervous system, and opposes the effect of adrenalin.

People with moderate to severe growth hormone deficiency often feel overwhelmed, anxious, and powerless. They have poor resistance to stress. They are nervous and irritable. Even if they have a full night's sleep, they do not feel restored in the morning. Administration of growth hormone leads to a decrease in the need for sleep and a better night's rest.

Growth hormone helps with concentration and attention, self-confidence, and the ability to find solutions for problems.

Factors that stimulate secretion of growth hormone include testosterone and DHEA, estrogen, L-DOPA, nicotine, arginine, the blood pressure medications propranolol and clonidine, insulin, deep sleep, niacin, vigorous exercise.

Factors that lower growth hormone levels include high blood sugar, cortisol and similar hormones (prednisolone and dexamethasone), DHT, and medications such as phenothiazines.

It has been found that 80% of people who have had a head injury, especially with a loss of consciousness, suffer from growth hormone deficiency, apparently due to trauma to the pituitary gland. Everyone who has had a concussion should be tested for growth hormone deficiency.

Growth hormone should be replaced only under the supervision of an experienced physician—and only with documented GH deficiency. Unnecessary or improper administration of growth hormone can result in serious side effects, some of which may be irreversible. These include carpal tunnel syndrome, the elevation of blood sugar, diabetes, excessive growth of internal organs (brain, liver, kidneys, and lungs) thickening of the skin, and growth of chin, nose, ears, and supraorbital ridges.

Properly administered replacement therapy in deficient patients results in improved appearance, younger look, weight (fat) loss, increase in lean body mass, improvement of metabolic syndrome, increase in mental and physical performance, and improved self-esteem.

Many questions remain unanswered regarding the relationship between growth hormone replacement and cancer. Some studies show that higher growth hormone increases the incidence and accelerates the spread of some cancers, while others show opposite results.

No one with a history of cancer should, in my opinion, use growth hormone, but those who suffer from severe growth hormone deficiency should seriously consider GH replacement therapy.

Chapter 17

Appetite Regulation

As we already know, every living organism is an open system. It receives energy and substance in the form of food from the environment, uses it to maintain life functions, and returns it in the form of heat and substances (body tissues and waste).

This system is most stable in a steady state—when it receives just as much energy and substance as it needs to spend. Ideally, after completion of growth, energy intake and expenditure should be equal.

This, unfortunately, is not the case. After maturation, the fat mass in the organism starts to increase. Why does this happen?

This phenomenon may be explained by the fact that animals are not just machines that work by the laws of physics and chemistry. We cannot "get rid" of biological laws in order to not lose the ability to develop and thus to live.

While growing and developing, we need a lot of food—especially proteins and fats—to build a body from a 7-pound newborn to a 160-pound male or 130-pound female. But what happens after growth stops? Our appetite is supposed to significantly decrease due to our decreasing requirements for energy and substance. However, this does not happen. Our appetite does not decrease, and this leads to an increase in the fat content of the body.

The most common explanation for this increase in fat mass is that with age, a person starts to have less physical activity. But this explanation is only valid if there is a significant decrease in physical exercise or a significant increase in food consumption.

But everyone remembers when they were 20 to 25 years old. Weight was generally stable despite changes in physical activity and the amount of food eaten. This proves that there is a mechanism of regulation of body weight—either by controlling the amount of energy entering the body as food or by regulating the release of energy as heat.

Currently, regulation of appetite has been more thoroughly researched than regulation of energy release.

It seems very simple. Suppose the weight of the body is controlled. In that case, appetite should tightly correspond to the amount of energy spent, and if physical activity decreases with age, so should the appetite.

In reality, however, this does not happen.

It is simple to measure the amount of energy that enters the body, like an electric meter in your house. But it is impossible to keep an accurate record of the energy you have expended.

So, what do we know now about appetite regulation in the body?

We know that it consists of two different mechanisms.

The first mechanism corrects the amount of fat in the organism, indirectly, by controlling the level of insulin, the pancreatic hormone necessary for transporting glucose into cells. The concentration of insulin is correlated tightly with fat mass in the body. If the fat mass in the body increases, the insulin level increases correspondingly. The hypothalamus detects this increase in insulin, and a series of reactions is triggered to decrease the fat mass, and thereby the insulin level. This mechanism can be called the "strategic center of appetite" because it regulates processes that take a long time to implement.

The second hypothalamic mechanism controls the concentration of energetic substances in the blood, mainly glucose. But this one measures the amount of fuel (glucose and possibly fatty acids) during each meal. Therefore, it can be called the "tactical center of appetite."

Furthermore, this tactical center of appetite consists of two hypothalamic centers: the food center and the satiation center.

When food is not being digested, the level of glucose is decreasing. This activates the food center of appetite to seek food. As a result, glucose and insulin levels increase. At a certain level, glucose stimulates the satiation center, which leads to a feeling of fullness. Simultaneously, the satiation center sends a signal to suppress the food center.

But even though classical medicine has already discovered how appetite is regulated, it does not explain why it gets disturbed. In an experiment, scientists destroyed the center of satiation in animals, and this resulted in increased appetite. But there is no evidence that the satiation center is destroyed when animals reach the age of maturity. Furthermore, at a very advanced age, appetite gradually diminishes. Also, appetite can change depending on many conditions, for example, when depressed, under stress, or even during extreme happiness.

So, what is the reason for the disruption of hypothalamic control of appetite with advanced age?

The study showed that the hypothalamus becomes less sensitive to the effect of glucose. The same amount of sugar in food causes a greater increase in blood sugar with aging. Because it is the rise of blood sugar that activates the center of satiation and inhibits appetite, so a feeling of fullness should appear faster rather than slower. This, however, does not happen, meaning that the satiation center is becoming less sensitive to the rise of glucose.

This is the reason why aging people need to eat more food for the satiation center to respond. Excess glucose that is not burned in the muscular tissue turns into fat, increasing insulin levels.

The strategic center that regulates the amount of fat should, in this case, respond to the increasing level of insulin and decrease it, thereby decreasing the amount of fat in the body. This occasionally occurs in young men when body mass increases through overeating—appetite decreases, and the body recovers to its initial mass. However, this does not happen in an aging man whose body mass increases in a step-like manner. There are periods when body mass increases and then remains stable for a while, as if a set point (or sensitivity of a regulator) in the strategic center changes.

Thus, changes in both strategic and tactical regulators of appetite are driven by the decreasing sensitivity of negative feedback mechanisms. What can explain the change in sensitivity?

In experiments, an artificial decrease in concentration of neurotransmitters in the hypothalamus—just as happens naturally with aging—leads to an increase in appetite.

And this is why, during a state of stress, when the need for neurotransmitters increases, younger people lose their appetite, but older people increase their appetite, indicating a lack of neurotransmitters.

Similarly, food intake can affect mood. A good meal usually improves mood, and this is because digesting a good meal—especially consisting of meat or fowl—increases the concentration of amino acids, the building blocks of protein. These amino acids include tryptophan, which converts to serotonin, a neurotransmitter that improves mood and stimulates the center of satiation.

On the other hand, the consumption of sweets (or sugar in any form), also improves mood. This is because rising glucose levels cause insulin to be released, and insulin contributes to the supply of tryptophan to the brain.

We can conclude that age-related dysregulation of appetite is just as common an occurrence as menopause. Both occur due to age-related sensitivity decreases in regulating centers in the hypothalamus.

An influx of energy is vital to the existence of an organism. However, once the energy influx escapes normal regulation by the hypothalamus, it becomes the main reason that most of the normal age-related diseases, such as diabetes and atherosclerosis, develop.

Chapter 18

Age-Related Obesity

It is well known to scientists that the fat content of the body increases with age.

Even if our overall bodyweight does not increase, the percentage of fat increases as we age, offset by a decrease in lean body mass. We need to distinguish between age-related obesity and non-age-related obesity, a disease in people who overeat and under-exercise.

A typical lean adult man who weighs 150 pounds has 20 pounds of fat in his body, so a 20-pound increase in weight corresponds to double the amount of fat.

Compare this to other parameters of the body—like blood pressure or blood sugar. A two-fold increase in blood pressure or blood sugar would represent a severe form of high blood pressure or diabetes.

Why does body fat mass increase with age? Most people attribute age-related obesity to a decrease in physical exercise in older people; however, this is not exactly correct. It only applies if intake of food significantly increases or physical activity decreases due to age-related issues.

However, most people can remember a time in their lives when, despite changes in food intake and physical activities, their weight remained relatively stable for years. This means that there are some mechanisms in the body responsible for the stabilization of body weight.

These regulatory processes can influence body mass by controlling the influx of energy in the form of food intake (appetite) or by regulating heat production and transfer in the body (temperature).

Fat mass regulation is impaired with aging due to the loss of sensitivity of the hypothalamus to changes in glucose and insulin. It is also a sign of loss of self-regulation and stability in the principal system of an organism—the energy homeostat.

Energy is the basis for existence of any organism, but when energy escapes regulatory control, it is responsible for the onset of major diseases.

This is why it is so important to understand mechanisms that control energy exchange, and like other self-regulation in the body, it is, of course, an interplay of hormones.

There are four major participants in this process:

1. *Growth hormone (GH)*
1. *Insulin (I)*
1. *Glucose*
1. *Fatty acids*

After a baby is conceived, tremendous amounts of building materials and energy are needed to support the rapid growth and development of the body. Millions of new cells need to be created every day. Each cell has a membrane made of cholesterol and special fatty acids. Cholesterol is made from energy-rich fat. The building process itself is energy-consuming and is powered by the burning of sugar and fat.

Growth continues until the time of sexual maturation, when growth of the body significantly slows down, around 18 years of age, and stops around age 25.

The daily process of growth and metabolism occurs in two phases: daytime and nighttime.

During the day, a child consumes fats and sugars as a source of energy. We always are amazed at how much children eat, especially sweet stuff. Isn't ice cream, a mix of fat and sugar, a children's favorite treat?

A large part of the sugars that they eat is burned in muscles due to a very high level of physical activity.

All excess sugars that are not burned in the muscles during the day are converted to fats in the liver and are saved for later use in the fatty tissue under the influence of insulin.

This type of energy production can be called "daytime metabolism" or "glucose-based metabolism".

At night, when the child sleeps, energy consumption is minimal; this is when most of the growth occurs.

A child sleeps a long time at night—10 or 11 hours—and does not eat during these hours. A long time of fasting causes a drop in blood sugar levels. This drop in blood sugar triggers the release of GH from the pituitary gland.

As we already know, GH has strong fat-mobilizing action. It moves fatty acids, which were accumulated throughout a day, from fatty tissue into the bloodstream.

Here we need to explain that unlike sugar, which needs insulin to get inside a cell to be burned, fatty acids easily penetrate through cell membranes, and their availability as energy supply is only determined by their concentration in the blood.

Thus, muscles are supplied with fatty acids as a preferred food substance, and sugar is saved for the brain tissue, which requires glucose as its main source of energy. At the same time, growth hormone causes the liver to produce growth-promoting IGF-1. Using fats that were accumulated throughout the day, the liver produces cholesterol for building the membranes of new cells.

So, we may call this type of energy production "nighttime metabolism" or "fat metabolism."

Here, negative feedback exists between GH and sugar levels—as soon as GH is released and blood sugar rises, secretion of GH ceases.

The same principle exists between GH and fatty acids, but this is through the participation of glucose. When fatty acid concentration increases and cells are supplied with energy, the consumption of sugar decreases. The resulting increase of blood sugar level stops the release of GH.

In childhood, due to the rapid growth and formation of new cells, there is increased demand for cholesterol which is synthesized from fatty acids. This is, apparently, the reason why fats themselves do not suppress GH levels in children. But in adults, who do not use so many fats for new cell membrane construction, fats have a much more pronounced effect in suppressing GH.

Upon reaching sexual maturity, the growth of the body slows down. This, along with decreased muscular activity compared to children, results in less demand for fatty acids, and their level in the blood starts to rise.

Being preferred food for muscles, fatty acids replace sugar as the main source of energy, not only at night but also during the daytime.

Their availability creates a surplus of food, and sugar is not being burned as it was in the growing stage. The excess sugar needs to be removed from the blood, and this is achieved by converting sugar into fat in the liver and fatty tissues, under the influence of insulin.

This shift creates a situation where sugars are not burned directly but are first converted to fats and burned only when there is a short supply of fatty acids, which is extremely rare. The only time it happens is when muscles are actively working and need a surplus of energy in addition to available fatty acids.

So, in effect, after reaching maturity, we gradually shift from daytime and nighttime metabolism to nighttime metabolism only, and the amount of fatty tissue starts to increase.

At this point, the blocking effect of sugar on the production of GH diminishes, and the effect of fatty acids increases.

In childhood, when an organism is growing, a high level of fatty acids coexists with high levels of growth hormone because the sensitivity of the hypothalamus to fatty acids is lower and high levels do not suppress the release of growth hormone. This guarantees enough material and stimulus for the construction of new cells. At the same time, glucose inhibits growth hormone release, which effectively controls the switch between nighttime and daytime metabolism.

As time passes by, glucose sensitivity declines, and it does not suppress growth hormone as effectively. At the same time, fatty acids more and more effectively suppress growth hormone release.

Thus, when the concentration of fatty acids in the blood increases, it causes more and more decline in growth hormone, and because fatty acids are almost always high in aging, the level of growth hormone is always low. Even a minimal surplus of calories leads to an inevitable development of increased fat mass, in other words, age-related obesity.

There is another important factor in this vicious cycle.

Obesity decreases the activity of the thyroid gland. The thyroid hormone regulates the speed of chemical reactions in the body. A decrease in thyroid activity results in lower body temperature, a sign that the burning process has been slowed and that the amount of excess fat and sugar is therefore increasing.

Age-related obesity cannot be looked at as an isolated, normal disease of aging.

As soon as obesity develops, it self-perpetuates and disturbs many processes in the body, leading to the development of many age-related diseases.

We now know that the number of fat cells in an adult organism does not increase, so an increase in fat leads to an increase in cell size, not number.

This increase in size leads to the larger surface of the cell membrane, but the number of insulin receptors stays the same, which leads to a diminished effect of insulin.

The body responds by increasing production of insulin to maintain steady blood sugar levels. Insulin transforms excess glucose into fat and prevents the body using fat as energy. This is why obese people experience an increased sense of hunger even when their bodies hold a lot of unused fuel.

Fat cells, though, have a limited capacity to store fat. When they become overloaded, their membranes become thinner, and they start to release more fatty acids into the bloodstream despite increased levels of insulin. These fatty acids are utilized as fuel to produce energy, blocking sugar from being utilized as energy. This sugar is converted to more fat, creating another vicious cycle.

The level of growth hormone declines in humans between age 20 and 39 which means that this process of fat accumulation begins at an early age, right after the body stops growing.

Gradually, as obesity develops and fat becomes a major source of energy, cells become less and less sensitive to the action of insulin. Sugar that does not get converted to fat accumulates in the bloodstream, which is diabetes.

At the same time, when the capacity of fat cells to store fat is exceeded, fat is consumed by phagocytes, white blood cells that are responsible for eating and digesting harmful particles such as bacteria. When overfilled with fat, these cells, called foam cells, are incapable of their normal defensive actions, thus causing a defect in the immune system.

Along with insulin, organisms produce insulin-like growth substances called somatomedins. An increased amount of these leads to the development of atherosclerosis and cancer.

Obesity contributes to the development of high blood pressure, which increases the speed of blood flow through the heart. This is necessary to supply a larger body with oxygen and nutrients.

Obesity increases the ability of platelets (the clotting cells) to glue together, which increases the probability of heart attacks and strokes.

Chapter 19

Atherosclerosis

Heart attacks and strokes are diseases that most people know about and fear. But they are the consequences of a normal disease of aging called atherosclerosis (*atheroma* meaning "fatty tumor", *sclerosis* meaning "hardening"). Popularly, it is called hardening of the arteries.

Atherosclerosis develops to some degree in each aging animal, and this is why it may be considered a normal disease of aging. It is closely related to changes in the energy homeostat brought on by aging. Cholesterol plays the main role in the development of atherosclerosis. It is well known that an increase in blood cholesterol leads to an accelerated development of the condition. Injuries to the inside wall of arteries brought about by inflammation, or some viruses, can lead to deposition of cholesterol in these areas to patch damaged surfaces. So, even without elevated cholesterol, atherosclerosis can develop in non-obese individuals.

As we now know, the evolution of the energy homeostat that is brought about by changes in insulin and growth hormone brings about the transition from a glucose-based energy exchange (day/night metabolism) to a fat-based one (night metabolism). That change results from the excessive use of fatty acids for energy production while extra glucose is being converted to triglycerides and cholesterol (fat) in the liver.

Triglycerides and cholesterol cannot be released by themselves into the bloodstream because, as fats, they would form fatty bubbles in the water-based bloodstream. Therefore, in the liver, they are first attached to special carrier proteins. The newly formed complexes are called lipoproteins; in this form, they are soluble in water and are released into the bloodstream as very low-density lipoproteins, or VLDL, to be transported into tissues.

Here, energetic and structural lipoproteins separate. Triglycerides are delivered into cells to supply energy, and cholesterol that is connected to protein forms low-density lipoprotein (LDL), which is used to make cell membrane structures.

Unused cholesterol is transported out of the cells into the blood in the form of high-density lipoproteins that then enter the liver and are expelled in the bile.

The density of lipoproteins is determined by the ratio between fats and proteins in lipoproteins.

The higher the protein content, the higher the density. HDL increases with an increase of physical exercise but decreases as age progresses.

Cell membranes have receptors that detect LDL and transport it inside the cells to supply building materials for new cell formation.

At an early age, when maximum growth and development occurs, large amounts of cholesterol are needed to meet the demand for building membranes of newly forming cells.

Younger organisms have a mechanism for decreasing cholesterol production by the liver if enough cholesterol is obtained in food.

This mechanism gradually becomes ineffective in the grown-up animal due to a decrease in the formation of new cells and thus the use of cholesterol.

A rising cholesterol level in the bloodstream provides an abundant source of cholesterol for cells in the inner surface of blood vessels. These cells still retain an ability to divide, and excess cholesterol, in the presence of an increased level of anabolic insulin, serves as a stimulant for division.

There is a theory that atherosclerotic plaque originates from a single smooth muscle cell in a blood vessel wall. This cell is stimulated to divide because of the abundance of cholesterol. As a result, a plaque consisting of elements of muscular and connective tissues, saturated with cholesterol and impairing the free flow of blood, is formed.

In addition, free fatty acids have the ability to increase clot formation in the blood, which creates perfect conditions for the formation of a blood clot in the vicinity of plaque.

The development of atherosclerosis is another example of a vitally important mechanism of new cell formation that, when working erroneously and in excess, is transformed into one of the major diseases of aging.

There is another major effect of increased fats in the body. This one affects the immune system.

Chapter 20

Fat-Induced Immunodepression

In the previous chapter, we briefly touched on a mechanism that the body employs to protect itself from excess cholesterol. HDL, which is formed when excess cholesterol is detected inside the cell, is subsequently expelled into the bloodstream to be transported to the liver. It is then expelled by the liver, as a component of bile, into the gut. However, there is another mechanism that may be used to get rid of cholesterol—the immune system.

The immune system is the organism's system of defense against invaders. This defense is carried out by special groups of white blood cells, namely lymphocytes and macrophages.

Lymphocytes are divided into two major groups: B lymphocytes, which produce antibodies, and T lymphocytes, which can directly kill cancer cells and cells infected with viruses.

Macrophages are white blood cells that are also called "janitor cells" because they are able to engulf and digest anything that they consider non-self, including cancer cells, microbes, cellular debris, foreign substances, and others.

Lymphocytes circulate throughout the body, seemingly doing nothing—like police cars on patrol. They are born, develop, and die like any other cells. But as soon as they detect an enemy, something that has a protein they are unfamiliar with, they undergo certain changes and acquire the capacity to multiply, just like becoming young again. Every newly formed T lymphocyte soon acquires the ability to divide. The army of T lymphocytes attack and kill invaders and continue dividing until the enemy is defeated. Just like any unicell, the lymphocyte depends on its external environment for survival, and just like amoebas, they die when changes in the external environment exceed their ability to adapt. If an amoeba's habitat is the pond, the lymphocyte's habitat is the bloodstream that provides an unlimited amount of food.

Increased fatty acids, cholesterol, and insulin may act as toxins to lymphocytes, if present in abnormally high concentrations.

In addition, lymphocytes, like all other cells, receive cholesterol in the form of LDL. When a lymphocyte circulates for a prolonged time in blood with high LDL content, excess cholesterol is accumulated on its membrane, making it less pliable and impairing its sensitivity to signals from enemies and its ability to divide.

This leads to a decrease in immune system response and exposes the organism to unnecessary dangers.

On the other hand, macrophages, too, consider fatty particles as toxic and engulf them. But their ability to digest is limited, and they accumulate undigested fat inside the cell. If they are too full of fats, they will be unable to render defense when needed.

On top of this, an increased level of insulin in the blood leads to a decrease in the number of insulin receptors on the lymphocyte's surface and a decrease in response to the glucose-mobilizing action of insulin. This moves the lymphocyte from glucose-based energy to dangerous fatty acid-based energy, further impairing its defensive potential.

This is how elevated fats in the bloodstream cause the depression of immune system responses, which can be called fat-induced immunodepression.

Chapter 21

Adrenaline, Epinephrine, and Norepinephrine

Bobby and his girlfriend Ann went to a sports bar to have a drink and a bite to eat. They ordered their drinks and had just taken a first sip when a drunken man approached them and unceremoniously grabbed Ann's arm and started trying to drag her to his table.

Bobby jumped up from his chair, blood rushing to his head. He was breathing heavily and veins on his neck bulged. His heart was pounding, his legs were shaking, and he had goosebumps. He was full of rage and ready to throw the first blow to the offender's jaw. All this happened within a split second—he did not even have time to think.

Bobby was under the influence of the hormone adrenaline. The hormone of fear, fight, and flight.

Adrenaline and epinephrine, like noradrenaline and norepinephrine, are interchangeable names for important hormones produced in the central part of the adrenal gland and the brain.

The word "adrenaline," which is used in the United Kingdom and Europe, derives from Latin roots, *ad* meaning "at" or "near" and *ren* meaning "kidney". In the United States we use the same words but in Greek: *epi* meaning "above" and *nephros* meaning kidney. So, we will adhere to epinephrine for now.

Epinephrine was first isolated in 1895 by polish physiologist Napoleon Cybulski.

In 1901, Japanese chemist Jokichi Takamine patented a purified extract from adrenal glands and called it Adrenalin. It was trademarked, and the European Pharmacopeia term for this drug is Adrenalin. However, pharmacologist John Abel had already produced a similar extract in 1897 and coined the name epinephrin. The notion that Takamine's and Abel's extracts were identical is now being disputed. However, the names of receptors and classes of medications that pertain to adrenaline are called adrenergic.

Epinephrine is synthesized in the adrenal medulla (the central part) of adrenal glands, from the essential amino-acid phenylalanine or the non-essential amino-acid tyrosine. Phenylalanine is converted to tyrosine, then tyrosine is converted to DOPA, DOPA is converted to dopamine, dopamine is converted to norepinephrine, and norepinephrine is converted to epinephrine. These three substances (dopamine, norepinephrine, and epinephrine) are called catecholamines, and all three are neurotransmitters.

However, norepinephrine and epinephrine are also hormones with similar, but not identical, actions. We are not talking here about dopamine because it is a neurotransmitter and not a hormone.

Norepinephrine and epinephrine are stress hormones of immediate response, and that means their function is to modify all target organs in a way that is more conducive to active body state during stressful situations (fight or flight) at the expense of higher energy use and increased wear and tear.

They are released within a split second following an electrical nerve impulse from the central nervous system, and their action precedes the slower action of cortisol, the steroid stress hormone.

They increase heart rate and blood pressure to increase circulation and the supply of oxygen and nutrients to muscles, heart, lungs, and brain. They cause a rise in blood glucose by converting animal starch, which is stored in the liver for just these occasions, into sugar. They increase the speed of mental processing and muscle strength, and suppress inflammation and the immune system, actions that are beneficial at the time of stress. They also redistribute blood from digestive and sex organs to muscles, lungs, heart, and brain. They make muscles shake, a sign that they are ready for action.

In short, epinephrine and norepinephrine, within a split second, achieve the change which takes athletes 30 to 45 minutes to warm up to prior to performance in a competition. In other words, they create a storm in the body.

The action of norepinephrine and epinephrine is very short-lived. Their half-life in the blood is only 3 to 4 minutes. By that time, the cortisol that was released in the blood is simultaneously starting to work, performing very similar functions but on a more sustainable energetic basis.

In addition to their role as hormones, norepinephrine and epinephrine are very important excitatory neurotransmitters. They facilitate the transmission of signals in the nervous system, where their actions are similar but not identical. Amphetamines and appetite suppressants exert a norepinephrine-like effect on the brain.

Norepinephrine, aside from its excitatory action, also has regulating qualities, while epinephrine is purely excitatory.

Epinephrine is implicated in the development of long-term memory for stressful events, and the more stressful the event was, the more deeply it is imprinted in the brain. An animal will use these memories in the future when exposed to similar threats. It is an important factor in the development of PTSD as well.

Norepinephrine, on the other hand, is antidepressant and an activator of mental alertness.

Medications that increase norepinephrine in the brain are used to treat depression, attention deficit hyperactivity disorder (ADHD), and as appetite suppressants.

Epinephrine is used as medicine for acute allergic reactions and in the management of shock. It is injected when antiallergic action is needed within seconds, as in the case of an anaphylactic reaction, an overwhelming allergic reaction that may lead to death within minutes if untreated. People who are allergic to bee stings or peanuts carry an Epi-Pen, to self-inject epinephrine at the first sign of an allergic reaction. Cortisol is also used for a similar purpose, but only if the action could be postponed for 20 to 30 minutes.

Chapter 22

Cortisol

X thought that something was wrong with him. After a traumatic divorce followed by the death of his mother, he felt that life had changed. He started to lose weight, his face became thin, and his cheeks grew hollow.

He lost energy and felt tired all day long but especially after lunch around 2 to 3 p.m. His energy would eventually get better after an hour or so, but fatigue would return around 7 p.m.

His doctor was surprised to see that his blood pressure, which had been borderline-high before, became low, and his blood sugar dropped to the lowest reference range.

He developed sugar cravings and a liking for very salty food. His joints and muscles became achy all over his body. He started to suffer from allergies. His skin became somewhat darker, especially on the lines of his palms.

Usually very agreeable, he became cranky and started to blame everyone for his misfortunes and mistakes. At the same time, he became extremely compassionate even at his own expense and could not abstain from offering help to others. He frequently shed a tear, especially watching touchy movies. His body felt inflamed all over, and life did not feel like it was worth living.

XX was suffering from cortisol deficiency. So-called "adrenal fatigue," a term coined by James Wilson, an American doctor who described chronic insufficiency of the adrenal glands that was not severe enough to be called a disease.

MT was one of twins. Both were petite and slender European women, 4 feet, 11 inches tall. Like most identical twins, they were almost impossible to distinguish from one another.

At a certain point in her life, MT started to gain weight. She went for her yearly checkup and found out that she had very high blood pressure and high blood sugar. Her family doctor prescribed blood pressure medication and told her to stay on a diet, but it did not help. Blood pressure medication was doubled, but to no avail.

After a span of only one year, she no longer looked like her twin sister at all. She had a round face with red cheeks. She gained weight, but it was only in the middle of her body. Her legs thinned. She needed to take three blood pressure medications, but it remained uncontrolled, and her blood sugar rose, which required medicine as well. She was diagnosed with three conditions, obesity, high blood pressure, and diabetes.

She continued to be very vivacious—probably even more than before—but worried about her blood pressure. She decided to seek advice from her friend, a functional medicine doctor, who recommended a check of her cortisol level, which tested very high. After a series of tests, she was found to have a cyst in her adrenal gland that was producing excessive amounts of cortisol.

The cyst proved to be benign and was removed. Her cortisol returned to normal, and within months she lost all excess weight; her blood pressure returned to normal even without medication, and her blood sugar also dropped to low normal levels. In another year, she again became indistinguishable from her twin sister, something they had both hated since early childhood.

MT can serve as an example of cortisol excess.

Cortisol was discovered in the 1930s by Edward Kendall, Tadeus Reichstein, and Philip Hench as one of several compounds derived from adrenal glands.

Cortisol is produced in the outside layers (cortex) of the adrenal glands.

Its level is controlled by adrenocorticotropic hormone (ACTH) from the pituitary, which in turn is controlled by corticotropin-releasing hormone from the hypothalamus.

It is a vitally important hormone. Even though it is called the "stress hormone," cortisol is a life-sustaining hormone. An animal without a thyroid gland can survive for weeks and without sex glands for decades, but when adrenal glands are removed, death occurs within six to twelve hours due to a fatal drop of blood pressure to zero, unless cortisol is being supplemented.

Cortisol is produced in large amounts during the time of stress. It acts as a long-acting extension of epinephrine.

Cortisol is an adaptation hormone, meaning it is necessary to withstand stress, be it a fight or flight situation, rapid changes of temperature, infection, or other factors which necessitate adjustment. Even though the effects of increased cortisol may be detrimental in the long term, all of them are life-saving during a stressful situation. Probably the most accurate description of cortisol is "defense hormone."

Cortisol raises blood pressure which increases the supply of oxygen and nutrients to organs necessary for fight and flight situations such as the brain, heart, lungs, and muscles.

A very important function of cortisol is its effect on glucose metabolism. This is why hormones in this group are called glucocorticoids, in other words, hormones that are produced in the cortex of the adrenal gland which act on glucose. During fight or flight, there is no time to eat and replenish energy. All energetic resources have to come from within the body to feed muscles and the brain while they are working at maximum capacity. This is accomplished by a chemical process called gluconeogenesis, or in plain English, "new glucose generation".

It is a process where proteins of the body are converted into sugars. Usually, this does not occur except in situations of stress, and only happens during fight or flight when it is not possible to replenish energy by eating.

However, by converting protein, the most valuable substance in the body, into sugar, cortisol is causing loss of muscle and collagen, thus accelerating aging of the muscles, skin, and joints. It lowers bone formation, favoring the development of osteoporosis in the long term.

Cortisol not only stimulates gluconeogenesis but also decreases sensitivity to insulin which helps in maintaining higher levels of glucose. This action, however, contributes to the development of diabetes if exercised outside of fight or flight reactions, and when glucose is not burned by increased muscular activity.

It reduces inflammation and suppresses the immune system, actions which are beneficial during stress. This is also frequently utilized in the treatment of inflammatory, allergic, and autoimmune diseases such as rheumatoid arthritis, lupus, and asthma.

It stimulates gastric acid secretion to increase digestion but at the same time redistributes blood away from digestive organs, which can cause stomach ulcers and heartburn.

It cooperates with epinephrine (adrenaline) to create memories of short-term emotional events, which helps us remember dangers to avoid in the future—however, long-term exposure to cortisol results in impaired learning.

It shuts down the reproductive system which is not necessary during fight or flight.

This is why we lose sexual desire in stressful situations.

In an experiment, even rats whose cortical brains had been removed were able to become pregnant and give birth to offspring. But healthy young rats could not procreate when subjected to stressful stimuli.

Fertility returns when stress abates, after cortisol levels are reduced back to normal levels.

Chapter 23

Stress, the General Adaptation Reaction

S tress.

"I'm under stress." "I'm under *a lot* of stress." "I'm *so stressed!*"
How often do you hear it from people around you?

I hear it a lot.

I come into an examination room and see a nervous patient. Her muscles are tense. She cannot sit still. She grabs her phone, looks at the screen, and puts it down. She looks at her watch, changes her body position, looks at me, then at the phone screen again. Her movements are fast. Her blood pressure is slightly high, and her pulse is faster than normal. Her whole appearance emanates tension.

"How are you?" I ask.

"Oh, Doctor, I'm under so much stress."

Everyone knows what she means. Everyone has experienced that feeling.

But very few people know what "stress" really means, and few people realize that if they really understood what stress is, they would never want to get rid of it.

Without the ability to make a stress response, an animal cannot live for more than 6 to 12 hours. It dies from a fatal drop in blood pressure.

If used properly, the term stress describes a reaction of defense necessary to protect the life of an organism when the mobilization of all resources is necessary.

What people mean by being "under stress" is really a physical condition caused by the perception of danger, and the associated hormonal changes in response to this danger.

Whenever you need to rev up your energy to struggle for your life, you make stress. When the temperature rises, you need stress to cool your body down. When the temperature falls, you need stress to warm your body up.

When a virus or bacteria invades your body, you need stress to mobilize your body to fight it. You need stress to run away from the tiger or to fight an intruder who enters your house.

In other words, you need stress to mobilize all your defenses and maintain the stability of the body's internal environment.

It would probably be more effective to have a specific response to each of the different offending factors, but this would require a lot more complexity. This is why nature, in its infinite wisdom, created stress, a single basic reaction which the body employs to respond to any threat immediately and automatically. This reaction in the scientific language of biology is called the "general adaptation reaction" because it makes no difference what specific threat it responds to.

Later on, different mechanisms may be involved to address specific aspects of the threat, but in the beginning, we have no time to hesitate. We need to be prepared to fight for our life instantaneously.

Like everything else in the body, the general adaptation reaction is controlled by the neuroendocrine system, which is a hormonal reaction managed by the brain.

Hans Selye, a Hungarian scientist who developed a theory of stress has studied changes in the body caused by adverse influences. He is the one that called this condition *distress*, but just like we frequently use the word 'cause instead of *because*, people started to omit the first syllable and use the term stress instead of distress.

We need to remember that stress really means a reaction in response to changing circumstances which threaten to change our homeostasis, the stability of the internal environment, that is essential for saving life.

Let us see what happens in the body from a hormonal point of view during stress, using the well-known stressful situation of a dog meeting a cat.

A dog and a cat meet. Even at a distance, the sense organs detect an enemy and send signals to the central nervous system that an enemy is near; there is a possibility of a fight, and preparations must be made. Information is analyzed by the brain and sent to the hypothalamus, where emotions of fear and aggression are generated. It is the hypothalamus that mainly controls the generation of emotions. The cat assumes the typical pose, arching its back. The pose itself prepares an animal for immediate action. The dog also assumes a position of fear and aggression. His tail is tense, his hair is standing on its end on the withers, and his hind legs are tight.

At the same time, in both animals, the hypothalamus sends a signal through the sympathetic part of the autonomic nervous system. This signal momentarily reaches a part of the adrenal glands that produce adrenaline, the immediate stress hormone. You can easily see the action of adrenaline because it causes hair to stand on its end by contracting special muscles in the skin. The release of adrenaline causes redistribution of blood flow, redirecting it from skin, digestive, and sex organs to the brain, heart, lungs, and muscles. Only the organs that are needed during a fight should have beneficial treatment. This is why in stressful situations, our mouth gets dry, and occasionally, people have an uncontrolled bowel movement, which occurs because the digestive system is switching off. This is where the expression comes from, indicating that someone was extremely scared. An animal or person may have uncontrolled urination. In this case, the body turns off reproductive organs and gets rid of waste, which is extra weight and degrades ability for the best fight or flight.

Adrenaline also increases heart rate and raises blood pressure to better supply the brain, lungs, heart, and muscles with oxygen and nutrients, which is crucial during a fight.

Performing all these changes requires energy, and adrenaline releases sugars stored in the liver to increase energy supply to the brain and muscles for the first 3 to 4 minutes. This, together with trembling of the muscles, increases muscle temperature. Increased temperature indicates the speeding of chemical reactions, which is important for optimal performance. Within a split second, all these changes achieve complete readiness for stellar performance. However, the action of adrenaline only lasts 3 to 4 minutes because it is very rapidly destroyed in the bloodstream. But just in time, another system is ready to take over the stress response: simultaneous with the sympathetic signal in the first moment of stress, the hypothalamus had also sent a hormonal signal to the pituitary gland to release growth hormone, prolactin, and adrenal stimulating hormone (ACTH) and these are now circulating in the bloodstream.

Growth hormone and prolactin mobilize the release of fatty acids from fat depots into the bloodstream. Fat is a muscle's favorite food, and gives six times more energy than glucose. This influx of energy further increases body temperature. Prolactin also suppresses the production of FSH and LH by the pituitary to suppress the function of sex organs.

This hormonal action is needed because adrenaline is causing such a storm in the body that if stress is not short-lived, the body will simply run out of energy. It needs a more solid energy source.

At the same time, ACTH stimulates the release of cortisol, which has several functions.

Cortisol has the ability to stimulate the conversion of protein into sugar to provide fast energy following the first minutes of fight or flight. Protein is the most precious material in the body, but during stress, when the life of the animal is on the line, this action is justified. Protein that is used in this instance needs to be unnecessary during a fight and be easily replaceable afterward. This is why immune white blood cells are first used for this purpose. They will be easily replaced by bone marrow later. We all know how easy it is for a person suffering from negative emotions and extreme stress to contract a cold because immunity has been weakened.

At the same time, it is beneficial to suppress the immune system during a fight because there will be damage to the tissues, and small particles of damaged skin, muscle, and other tissues may get into the bloodstream and be recognized by the immune system as foreign. In this case, an allergy to your own body, an auto-immune disease, could develop.

This is why cortisol, and its analogs prednisolone, dexamethasone, and others are used in the treatment of lupus, asthma, and other allergic and auto-immune diseases.

Aside from that, cortisol suppresses inflammation. Inflammation makes injuries more painful, and a wounded animal will be able to fight better with less pain, thus improving its chances of survival.

Growth hormone, prolactin, and cortisol also cause blood to clot more readily, which is protective during a fight (reducing blood loss from wounds)—but it can contribute to the development of heart attacks or strokes if it continues for a long time.

But at the time of a fight, everything that hinders the ability to fight, and to mount a successful stress reaction, has to be inhibited in order to save a life.

But now the fight is over. The animal is exhausted. It lies down and rests, unable to mount another fight or flight reaction. Pulse rate and blood pressure go back to normal. Blood is redistributed from brain, heart, lung, and muscle back to its normal, whole-body circulation, again supplying digestive and sex organs.

Neurotransmitter levels need some time to be restored, and this is why an animal is in a state of stupor, called a refractory period. After some time, when neurotransmitters return to low-normal levels, the animal exits the refractory state.

Excess fatty acids in the blood that were used to raise temperature and feed the muscles during stress are used to make the cholesterol necessary for rebuilding cell membranes and repairing tissues damaged during the fight. This is why cholesterol increases after stress.

Here is an interesting question that needs to be answered.

Why does the release of cortisol continue throughout the duration of the fight—why is it not under the control of negative feedback? The answer is that during a fight, neurotransmitters are used in enormous amounts, to such a degree that the hypothalamus loses sensitivity to cortisol and does not suppress releasing factor even though levels are higher than normal.

This sensitivity is partially restored when neurotransmitters return to normal levels after the refractory phase.

We need to remember that the stress reaction, as it is described above, is initiated not only when you encounter an enemy, but also any time when the hypothalamus determines that you need an immediate adaptation to any harmful factor, be it a bacterial infection, rapid change of temperature, or even when you are late for an appointment, which is perceived as danger.

Nature, in its wisdom, does not differentiate between these situations. These reactions are initiated every time you need to rev up the defense. This is why it is called a *general* adaptation reaction—and not just an adaptation reaction.

Of course, all these changes come at great expense to the organism—but when survival is on the line, it is definitely justified.

Hans Selye, the author of the theory of stress, studied this phenomenon for decades. In his laboratory, he stressed animals to death, studying all of the associated processes. On autopsy, these animals all showed stomach ulcers and bruises in the adrenal glands. They all developed high blood pressure and diabetes.

When an animal is in a state of distress, the production of cortisol increases several-fold, and most of the pregnenolone gets used up in making so much cortisol. This results in a decrease in the production of other steroid hormones, especially sex hormones which, together with prolactin, turns off the reproductive system.

This is why animals and humans have no sex drive at the time of stress.

As we have seen, stress is an extremely important mechanism of defense, but when the reserve of the adrenal glands is exceeded, and an animal is not able to mount an adequate stress reaction, it can die in response to minimal changes in its external or internal environment.

This is why it is so important to reserve the general adaptation reaction only for incidents of real danger—and take life easy the rest of the time.

And this leads us to the topic of chronic stress.

Chapter 24

Hyperadaptosis

In the previous chapter, we discussed the development of the general adaptation reaction or stress.

Here we will talk about age-related changes in the adaptation homeostat, which is somewhat different from development of the reproduction and energy exchange homeostats.

We sometimes hear from patients that their parents died from old age, especially if it happens after the age of 80. They may not be diagnosed with any of the diseases of aging such as diabetes, high blood pressure, heart attacks, atherosclerosis, or cancer—yet they suddenly die, with no known cause or disease, often in their sleep. That is when it is said that they died from old age.

But old age by itself cannot be a cause of death—there is still some reason why they died at that certain point in their life. If there was no cause, they would have continued living.

It is a well-known expression that any chain is as strong as its weakest link, so there must be some weak link that causes death in these people.

We know that anabolic hormones, testosterone, estradiol, progesterone, growth hormone, DHEA, and pregnenolone all start to decline in the fourth decade of human life, leading to gradual decline and dysregulation of the energy and reproduction homeostats. But one hormone, namely cortisol, goes the opposite direction, and its level continues to increase past the age of 30.

Why does cortisol not follow the other hormones and decline with age too? And what is the significance of this phenomenon?

Before answering that question, we need to revisit a related question we answered in the previous chapter: Why during fight or flight does cortisol escape the regular influence of the negative feedback mechanism and continue being released until the fight is over?

During stress, just like at any other moment, rising cortisol levels are supposed to initiate a decline in the production of releasing factor from the hypothalamus and thus the release of ACTH, a pituitary hormone that stimulates the production and release of cortisol, thus maintaining homeostasis.

But this does not happen during the time of stress—cortisol is produced in large amounts until the fight is over.

The answer why this happens lies in the hypothalamus itself.

From the very first moment of encounter with an enemy and for the duration of the fight, extreme emotions of fear and aggression cause neurotransmitters in the hypothalamus to be used in much larger quantities than in normal situations. Neurotransmitters are necessary for nerve cells to transmit signals from one to another. It may be assumed that due to increased utilization, the hypothalamus simply runs out of neurotransmitters and cannot exercise the normal negative feedback suppressing the release of cortisol.

After mounting the defense mechanism, and if death is avoided either by winning a fight or successful escape, an animal enters a period of restoration, called the refractory period. Body temperature, elevated during stress by intensive burning of fatty acid, gradually declines.

Heart rate, speed of breathing, and blood pressure slowly return to normal, blood flow to digestive and sex organs gradually increases, brain activity slows down, and the animal enters an almost stuporous state until neurotransmitter levels in the brain are restored.

It is a period when the hormonal and energetic storm associated with stress subsides, and processes of restoration and repair take place.

After some time, the animal returns to the state of normalcy and continues to live as if nothing happened—until the need for a general adaptation reaction arises again.

During aging, the adaptational system is continuously bombarded by stress factors that demand activation of the system of protection. This increases the working capacity of the adaptation homeostat, which is evident in the increased level of cortisol.

However, when the hypothalamus becomes less sensitive to cortisol, it starts to operate with a lag. Cortisol levels do not return to prestress levels as fast, thus creating overall higher cortisol levels which gradually increase with aging. This mechanism is easily confirmed by the experiment we discussed in the chapter on homeostasis.

Recall that dexamethasone, a derivative of cortisol, has the same effect on the hypothalamus as cortisol, but it does not interfere with cortisol blood tests. A certain dose of dexamethasone is given to an animal. Blood is tested for cortisol before and after the injection. The cortisol level decreases after administration of dexamethasone due to negative feedback on the hypothalamus and pituitary gland.

For an equal dose of dexamethasone given to two animals, the amount of decline in cortisol level will depend on how sensitive the animal's hypothalamus is to the negative feedback action of cortisol. For example, cortisol level decreases by 51% in 2-month-old rats but only by 11% in 8-month-old rats.

We see the same effect in humans—cortisol level declines by 33% in 50-year-olds and by 47% in 35-year-olds.

The less sensitive the hypothalamus becomes, the more cortisol is needed to block stimulation of the pituitary gland, and the higher the level of cortisol will be in non-stressful situations. The condition develops when an organism is always living in a condition of stress, with increased blood sugar level, elevated blood pressure, decreased blood supply to sex and digestive organs, thinning muscles, and suppressed immune system.

At the same time, whenever an organism needs to mount a general adaptation reaction, the adrenal glands gradually become unable to increase the production of cortisol to the level necessary to mount the defense.

This is why in older age our ability to defend our internal environment declines, and even a minimal change in external or internal environment may prove deadly for older people.

So, "death from old age" is probably a death from an event that exceeds the reserves of the general adaptation homeostat, no matter how minor this event may be.

Chapter 25

Cancer

Each of the 30,000,000,000,000 cells in our bodies divides, just like the paramecium, leaving a progeny of 2. At the same time, cells are dying or committing cellular suicide (apoptosis). These two processes go on continuously throughout the life cycle. On average, every seven years, all cells are renewed, and no one cell is present in your body that was alive seven years ago. Over 3 million cells are born every second. All these cells are programmed to be valuable members of the body as a society. However, some of these cells are born with genetic mistakes. You cannot make billions and billions of births without any birth defects.

Sometimes these birth defects manifest in a transition from a normal cell of the body, with a pre-programmed limited life span, into a potentially immortal one. This cell becomes similar to a unicellular organism without internal causes of death and can divide as long as its external environment can support its life cycle.

This is proven by an experiment where cancerous cells were transplanted from one organism to another and survived significantly longer than the organism in which they originated.

We can conclude that the mechanism of this transition is incorporated in the genetic code of the cell. This mechanism was a main interest of scientists researching the mystery of cancer. This research has led to the discovery of many factors capable of causing this transition.

It was proven that many chemicals can transform normal cells into cancerous ones. For example, tobacco smoke causes a 10-fold increase in the incidence of cancer in smokers.

The other types of factors that can cause cancerous transformation are physical—for example, radiation.

Scientists also proved that biological factors (certain viruses) were able to enter a cell's DNA to cause cancer.

This may lead to the conclusion that different factors influence the same elements inside the cell to convert a normal cell into a cancerous one.

Between the ages of 20 and 65 years, the incidence of cancer increases almost 100-fold. But it is an oversimplification to say that the increasing frequency of cancer with age is just a result of accumulating exposure to carcinogens (chemicals that cause cancer). This can be proven by the following fact.

To advance the study of cancer, researchers created special "cancer" lines of animals—in this instance, mice. By the 5th month of life, 71% of these mice developed cancer of the mammary gland. But when their caloric intake was reduced from 16 to 10 calories a day, not a single animal developed cancer by this age.

With the advancement of cancer research, there is increasing evidence that not only the length and intensity of exposure to carcinogens but also the general condition of an organism determines the chances of developing cancer.

It is well known from statistics that obesity increases the probability of all kinds of cancers in humans. For example, obesity increases the chances of cancer in smokers almost seven times. Why does this happen?

The most important characteristic of a cancer cell is that it divides uncontrollably, so any factor that accelerates the rate of division will increase the chance of the development of cancer, and vice versa.

Cells that lose the ability to divide will never develop cancer.

In order to divide, a cell needs to accumulate enough energy and building materials. Even though cell division is supposed to guarantee the transfer of genetic material from the nucleus of the mother cell to two daughter cells, the factor that determines the readiness to divide is the presence of a sufficient amount of cholesterol to form membranes of daughter cells. This is why cell division will occur more frequently in the presence of an ample supply of cholesterol, and the deficit of cholesterol will prevent the cell from dividing.

The other factor in cancer development is a decrease in the activity of anti-cancer immunity. Our immune system has a mechanism to protect us against foreign cells killing all cells that are not our own.

This is well demonstrated in the case of organ transplants. Transplanted organs would be rejected unless cell-mediated immunity is suppressed by special medications.

As we already know, T lymphocytes, the cells that execute cell-mediated immunity, are poisoned by high levels of cholesterol and fat, rendering them unable to effectively defend the body by killing the abnormal cancer cells.

Adrenaline and cortisol, the stress hormones, both suppress the function of the immune system. By undermining defenses in this way, chronic stress leads to an increased chance of developing cancer.

The energy system also plays an important role in the formation of cancerous tumors. It was discovered that cancer cells use 10 to 30 times more glucose than normal cells and produce 10 to 30 times larger amounts of lactic acid, a product of anaerobic energy production (fermentation).

In the presence of oxygen, in other words, with burning, energy is produced from glucose 18 times more efficiently than by fermentation. It is only when more energy is needed than can be produced by oxidation, like during a strenuous weight-lifting session, that the fermentation process is employed. The aches in the muscles after a workout is caused by the presence of an increased amount of lactic acid.

Unicellular organisms, such as bacteria and amoeba, remain in a passive state when food is scarce and actively divide when food is plenty. Most of the time, they are hungry and are able to survive by internalizing minuscule amounts of nutrients from the environment. When nutrients become more available, they start to divide.

The case of complex, multicellular organisms is different. There is always a lot of glucose present in the blood, but cell membranes are impenetrable to glucose except in the presence of insulin. Without this barrier, glucose would freely enter cells and they would be continuously and uncontrollably dividing, provided there remained an unlimited amount of glucose.

Scientists discovered that the transformation of a normal cell into a cancerous cell requires only one gene. One gene determines the production of one protein. One such protein had been isolated from a cancerous tumor. The function of this protein is to "insulinize" the cell or make it very sensitive to the action of insulin and insulin-like factors. This ensures the increased flow of glucose into the cell, enabling it to divide and making it similar to a single-celled organism that just eats and multiplies. Increased fermentation can be explained by the fact that this transforming protein increases the ability of the cell to ferment glucose but does not affect the ability to burn it. This leads to an increase in the production of lactic acid.

In summary, as time passes, the length of exposure to carcinogens (such as chemicals, radiation, and viruses) increases, leading to increased formation of abnormal or cancerous cells that have increased ability to utilize glucose.

After the process of growth and development is completed, the amount of fat content in the body increases, and the energy homeostat changes to mainly fat-based production of energy, with increased levels of fatty acids and cholesterol in the blood, providing enough raw material for building cell membranes. The level of glucose in the blood is also gradually rising. This creates favorable conditions for accelerated division of cells due to increased availability of energy.

Due to the fat-induced suppression of the immune system, the anti-cancer function of T lymphocytes declines, allowing more and more atypical cells to remain undetected and allowed to survive.

All these factors—increasing cancerogenic exposure, ample supply of energy and building materials, and weakening of immune response—create better conditions for development and growth of cancerous tumors with advancing age.

Chapter 26

DHEA

Dehydroepiandrosterone (de-hydro-epi-andro-sterone) is too long a word for most of us to pronounce—let alone remember—so most of us call this hormone by its abbreviation DHEA.

It was discovered by Adolf Butenandt and Leopold Ruzicka in the early 1930s, the same ones who discovered and isolated testosterone.

DHEA is the most abundant steroid hormone in the human body. Because we do not yet know its exact function (despite its abundance), it has not been considered an important hormone until recently.

DHEA is short-lived in the body. It only exists in free form for 1 to 3 hours before it is utilized or attached to sulfur to become DHEA-sulfate (DHEAS) by the liver. Because DHEAS has a much longer half-life of 10 to 20 hours, its concentration in blood is 250 to 500 times higher than DHEA. DHEAS is converted back to DHEA when the need for DHEA arises.

Most of DHEA, about 70%, is converted to DHEAS, but only 13% of DHEAS is converted back to DHEA.

The levels of DHEA are very high during the fetal stage but fall rapidly after birth and remain low until the onset of puberty. At this point, DHEA levels gradually rise and reach a peak in the 3rd decade of life, between 20 and 30 years of age. The concentration of DHEA is two times higher in men than in women. After age 30, DHEA rapidly declines, much faster than other steroid hormones, suggesting that mechanisms of DHEA formation are unique. Some studies show that the decline of DHEA and DHEAS appears to be associated with a rise in cholesterol levels and overall development of aging. Other studies demonstrate that higher DHEA and DHEAS levels are associated with lower morbidity in life.

DHEA has a profound effect on the human organism.

DHEA is a precursor (parent molecule) of testosterone and subsequently estradiol in the body. Most of these hormones are produced through conversion from DHEA, even though minor amounts are derived from the progesterone branch of the steroidogenic pathway. It is possible that the steep decline of DHEA after the 3rd decade of life is responsible for declining levels of sex hormones in later life. Even though adequate levels of DHEA are necessary for optimal levels of testosterone (which is extremely important), this is not the only role that DHEA plays in the organism.

DHEA has a significant effect on the nervous system.

It has been discovered that DHEA is synthesized de-novo in the brain and is an important neurosteroid. DHEA acts as an excitatory neurosteroid which means that it activates the nervous system by suppressing the action of GABA, an inhibitory neurotransmitter, and activating the action of NMDA, an excitatory one.

In addition, DHEA and DHEAS act as σ_1 (pronounced "sigma-1") receptor agonists in the brain. It has been shown that σ_1-receptor agonists are effective in alleviating learning and memory disorders, mental impairment, and neurodegenerative diseases, including Alzheimer's disease, Parkinson's disease, amyotrophic lateral sclerosis, multiple sclerosis, and Huntington's disease.

Many antidepressants, such as Aricept and Elavil, are σ_1-receptor agonists.

It was noticed that DHEA is useful in the treatment of depression in patients with Alzheimer's disease even though most antidepressants had been proven ineffective or only minimally effective in this condition.

DHEA plays a role in the synthesis of nitric oxide (NO).

Nitric oxide is a simple molecule—just one nitrogen atom and one oxygen atom. The discovery of the role of NO as a signaling molecule in the body and its crucial role in the health of the blood vessel function was found to be worthy of a Nobel Prize.

Nitroglycerin which converts to NO in the blood, has been widely used in medicine as the primary treatment for heart attacks and angina since World War I, when it was noticed that workers in the factories that produced dynamite, which is made of nitroglycerin, had surprisingly low numbers of heart attacks. It is NO generation in the blood vessels in the penis that is a primary mechanism of action of Viagra, Cialis, and similar drugs.

As a matter of fact, Viagra was initially developed as a drug to protect against heart attacks, but when studies showed that erection was one of the side effects, it was reclassified and sold as an erection medication.

NO is necessary for the health of the inner lining of blood vessels, providing protection from atherosclerosis and spasm.

DHEA increases NO synthesis in the endothelium, the inner lining of blood vessels, and its anti-atherosclerotic properties can be attributed to this effect. DHEA slows down the development of atherosclerotic plaques, which cause blockage of arteries.

Epidemiological studies have demonstrated an inverse relationship between DHEAS levels and cardiovascular disease in men over 50 years of age (Barrett-Connor et al., 1986).

DHEA has an effect in preventing and treatment of metabolic syndrome. It has been shown to improve levels of cholesterol, reduce abdominal obesity, and lower blood sugar by blocking an enzyme implicated in the development of metabolic syndrome. The same mechanism is involved in ameliorating the effects of increased levels of cortisol.

DHEA takes part in regulating the action of IGF-binding protein 1 (IGFBP-1), which reduces the chances of developing cancers.

DHEA's usefulness in regulating IGFBP-1 as a molecular target against cardiovascular disease or cancer appears obvious.

Levels of circulating DHEAS are correlated with longevity in both monkeys and men.

Symptoms of DHEA deficiency are very vague. A dislike of loud sounds, thinning of armpit and pubic hair, and flattening of the mons pubis (the fat pad of the pubic area) in women are some of them.

Chapter 27

Pregnenolone, the Mother of All Steroids

The conversion of cholesterol into pregnenolone is the first step in the synthesis of all steroid hormones. It only takes one chemical reaction to convert cholesterol into pregnenolone. Pregnenolone does not have specific symptoms of deficiency, but it is still a very important hormone because the production of all steroid hormones, sex hormones, cortisol, DHEA, and others, depends on the availability of pregnenolone.

Pregnenolone was first synthesized by Adolf Butenandt in 1934.

The main symptom of pregnenolone deficiency is forgetfulness because it is present in high concentration in the brain and is one of the neurosteroids, which means that in the brain, it plays an active role of neurotransmitter and can be produced there. The other feature of pregnenolone deficiency is that it is a mixed bag of the symptoms of deficiencies in all the adrenal and sex steroid hormones. This can be explained by the fact that there is no other chemical except pregnenolone, from which steroid hormones can be synthesized.

We will not list all the symptoms of the other hormone deficiencies since they are described in other chapters. But when a patient presents with multiple hormone deficiency symptoms, we need to look for pregnenolone as a cause.

Temporary pregnenolone deficit can be caused by severe stress and is called pregnenolone steal syndrome. During severe stress, an organism needs to significantly increase the production of the stress and defense hormone cortisol. Due to the limited supply of available pregnenolone, almost all of it is used for the production of cortisol, and there is just not enough pregnenolone left to produce adequate amounts of other steroids. This situation leads to decreased levels of sex and adrenal steroids other than cortisol. No wonder we lose sexual desire under the influence of stress.

Pregnenolone has several actions in the brain. It helps to restore damaged nerve cells after trauma or stroke. It improves the transmission of signals between nerve cells. It has a sedative effect on the brain by augmenting action of the sedating neurotransmitter GABA, which is similar to the effect of medications such as Xanax, Valium, and other benzodiazepines. It is thought to improve memory. Pregnenolone also opposes the effect of marijuana on the brain by acting on cannabinoid receptors.

Pregnenolone was used in the 40s and 50s as medication to treat rheumatoid arthritis, but with the introduction of more potent anti-inflammatory drugs, its use was discontinued.

Pregnenolone does not cause a significant increase in steroid hormones when taken by mouth. Instead, it is converted to some neuroactive metabolites, one of which (allopregnanolone) was recently approved for the treatment of postpartum depression.

Pregnenolone is very useful during the time of stress and has no contraindications to its use.

Chapter 28

Melatonin

M elatonin was isolated by dermatologist Aaron Lerner in the middle of the 20th century from the cow's pineal gland. Lerner and his co-workers initially did not realize the significance of their discovery. They were interested in some special substance from the pineal gland that lightened and darkened the skin of amphibians. They decided to name this newly discovered molecule melatonin (*mela* from melanin, the pigment in the skin; *tonin* from serotonin, the neurotransmitter it derives from).

Before their discovery, the pineal gland was considered an atavism (an ancestral structure without a function). The discovery of melatonin established the pineal gland as an important organ of the endocrine system.

Melatonin regulates circadian rhythms, which coordinate the release of hormones according to the time of the day. For example, ideal cortisol levels are high at 8 a.m., slowly decreasing and reaching a nadir at 4 to 5 a.m. Testosterone, on the other hand, is highest during sleep and lowest in the late afternoon.

Melatonin also regulates hibernation. For example, bears sleep throughout winter when nights are long, and wake up at the onset of spring when days are becoming longer.

By the same mechanism, melatonin regulates seasonal reproduction in animals that mate only during certain times of the year. Usually, these times correspond with increased chances of survival for offspring, such as availability of food and water, ambient temperature, or feeding cycles of predators.

These influences are achieved mostly by perceiving fluctuations in light and darkness.

In mammals, maximal production of melatonin occurs during the night, and this is why it is considered a chemical expression of darkness. During the light period of the day, the blue part of the spectrum inhibits melatonin production.

A feature that distinguishes the pineal gland from classic endocrine glands is that negative feedback is not considered a factor in melatonin production regulated by light and darkness, making it mostly independent of hypothalamic influence. Instead, the pineal gland has a regulating effect on the hypothalamus. The absence of negative feedback control makes the pineal an unconventional gland. There is also nothing in evolution that restricts melatonin production to the pineal gland. Invertebrates, plants—and even unicells that have no glands—produce melatonin.

These invertebrates need melatonin just like vertebrates because of its antioxidant properties. Melatonin is about 100 times more potent an antioxidant than vitamin E.

Melatonin is dual action, having both receptor-dependent and receptor-independent mechanisms.

It binds to receptors and exerts hormonal influences. But it also works as a receptor-independent substance as a most potent free radical scavenger.

And that is not all. Melatonin's receptor-dependent action works in 3 ways.

It works as a peptide hormone, attaching to receptors on the surface of the cell membrane as well as a steroid hormone penetrating through the cell membrane and attaching to the receptor in the nucleus. Recently, a third type of melatonin receptor was discovered in the cytosol, the jelly-like substance inside cells. At the sites of all three receptors, melatonin has different effects.

When melatonin attaches to cell membrane receptors, it affects seasonal reproduction, circadian rhythms, sleep promotion, and bone growth. It lowers blood pressure and temperature during sleep.

When it attaches to nuclear receptors, it modulates the immune system and regulates antioxidant enzymes.

In the cytosol, melatonin takes part in detoxification and intracellular enzyme regulation.

The receptor-independent action of melatonin is mostly due to its uniquely superb antioxidant activity. Not only is melatonin extremely potent by itself, but substances that are produced after reaction with free radicals also have the ability to be antioxidants.

This antioxidant action is amplified by the fact that melatonin easily penetrates the blood-brain and blood-testicular barrier and exerts its antioxidant action where most other antioxidants are unable to go. In addition to that, melatonin easily penetrates into the mitochondria, the cell energy generators, where most reactive oxygen and nitrogen species (free radicals) are produced.

When compared with new, synthetically produced mitochondria-targeting antioxidants such as MitoQ and MitoE, which are concentrated in mitochondria up to 500-fold higher than regular CoQ10, melatonin still performed better in reducing free radical damage to this organelle.

This receptor-independent mode of action protects from ionizing radiation, ultraviolet radiation, heavy metal and alcohol toxicity, drug toxicity, and ischemia of the heart and brain.

By several mechanisms, melatonin impedes the growth and ability to spread metastases of cancerous tumors and increases the effectiveness of anticancer therapy. This is why it is being used more and more frequently as an adjunct to anticancer therapy.

Melatonin concentration in blood is not a good way of measuring melatonin because its concentration in different organs and inside the cells is higher than in the serum, so blood tests are unreliable.

With advancing age, the production of melatonin gradually diminishes, so in the elderly, the nocturnal rise in melatonin is either greatly diminished or no longer exists. This results in disruption of the sleep–wake cycle, which is of great importance for general health. In addition, decreased production of melatonin contributes to the accumulation of oxidative stress, which results in tissue aging in the skin, eyes, brain, muscles, liver, etc. This also contributes to the progression of diseases that have free radical components, such as neurodegenerative disease, cardiovascular disease, and metabolic syndrome.

In order to improve sleep, melatonin is used in small doses. However, to exert its potent antioxidant and anticancer activities, pharmaceutical doses of melatonin need to be used.

To conclude this chapter on melatonin, I need to reiterate that research into this hormone is in its beginning stage, so we can expect many interesting discoveries.

Chapter 29

Is Aging a Disease?

I n recent years there has been increased interest and popularity in hormone replacement therapy or HRT. Millions of people around the world are using HRT to prolong the state of youthfulness. Although there are more and more proponents of these therapies in the medical community, the majority of physicians do not consider HRT to be health-promoting.

The common consensus is that if diseases are eliminated, death will occur due to natural causes—in other words, because of aging itself—and that hormone therapies are risky attempts to promote youthfulness at the expense of possibly shortening the life span.

In their mind, aging is a natural process of loss of functional capacity of an organism, and that if diseases would not develop, organisms will continue to live until the maximum life span of the species is achieved.

We know that the concept of aging does not apply to animals unless they are domesticated.

They die because of predators, hunger, disease, and trauma long before reaching old age. Humans did not do much better, with only a few reaching old age before advances in medicine were made, mostly in the area of treating infections.

The average life span in Europe in the 17th century was around 30 years of age.

Here we need to define two different parameters: average life expectancy and maximum life span.

An average life expectancy is how many years an organism is expected to live.

The maximum life span is based mostly on observation and records and is usually based on the longest time between birth and death of a member of a species.

In humans, the maximum life span is 122 years for women and 116 for men—or roughly 120 years.

In these cases, we usually say that very old people die from "old age," but it is very hard to imagine that life would just extinguish (just like fire when there is no more wood) even though they do not starve to death. There must be a reason why they die, just as when people die at the age of 50.

The question is whether we can separate these two phenomena, aging and diseases, or there is a general process of developing diseases with the flow of time.

Now we need to determine the concept of disease. As we know, nearly all parameters in the body—body temperature, oxygen level, the concentration of chemicals in blood and tissues, blood pressure—need to be maintained within certain, usually very narrow, ranges. Therefore, any stable disturbance of a parameter can be considered a disease, for example, doubling of body fat mass or blood pressure or sugar level (severe obesity, hypertension, and diabetes).

Hundreds of diseases are known to medicine, but only a few of them cause the death of 80% of older people. Heart disease causes 23% of all deaths, and strokes from atherosclerosis cause 6%. Diabetes contributes another 5%. Hypertension (high blood pressure) and cancer add another 21.7%. The other ones are autoimmune diseases, depression of the immune system, and psychological depression.

In our medical system, we are technically using a digital approach. We determine that if any parameter falls below the 5th percentile, or above the 95th percentile, it constitutes a disease. Otherwise, the person is healthy.

But let us take an example of blood sugar levels.

We know that after a certain age, the rate of use of glucose by muscular tissue diminishes. This is proven by a glucose tolerance test. A person is given a sugary drink with a known amount of sugar in it. Sugar levels are then measured in 30-minute intervals. As a person ages, his blood sugar rises higher and higher and continues to be elevated for a longer time than in a younger person. This means that an older person has a temporary disturbance in a standard parameter, in this case blood sugar, which constitutes a disease. These changes in blood sugar levels do not reach the classic definition of diabetes but can be called temporary diabetes. In medical terms, it is called glucose intolerance. At the same time, older people release more insulin into the bloodstream than younger people during the glucose tolerance test. Higher insulin leads to an increase of fat content of the body, which is called obesity. When these changes reach a certain point and blood sugar is elevated continuously, we call it diabetes. At the same time, even the abnormal glucose tolerance test meets the definition of disease because any change that leads to an increased probability of death is a disease.

The same thing can be said about changes in the function of adaptation. To test the adaptation homeostat, we use the dexamethasone suppression test, which consists of measurement of the level of cortisol before and after injection of the synthetic cortisol-like medication dexamethasone. Due to negative feedback, the level of cortisol declines after the shot. This decline is much more significant in young adults than in 40-year-olds, and this difference increases with age. This demonstrates the stable disturbance of central control of cortisol production which can technically also be called a disease, but it happens to every aging individual without exception.

But there is no particular disease in the medical sense that is causing this phenomenon. It is a normal occurrence that is becomes more pronounced after an organism reaches full development.

We can see this process in the development of menopause. Every woman reaches the state when her reproductive activity ceases, and it is only because all women undergo this change that it is not considered a disease.

Thus, when we talk about aging as a "normal process" we only mean that everyone undergoes aging. The majority of gerontologists, doctors who specialize in the treatment of the elderly, say that it is not possible to consider all humans "patients" after reaching a certain age. They, however, do consider premature aging as a disease.

But it is possible to see aging as a disease because it is a stable disturbance of homeostasis in the three major homeostats, namely energy, adaptation, and procreation.

The fact that changes occur simultaneously in many systems with multiple symptoms—and occur in everyone—does not make it a norm. In fact, it is the diversity and multitude of presentations of aging that is the main reason we consider it a norm, and the different constituents of this overall process like heart disease, cancer, diabetes, and others are considered separate diseases and not different presentations of a disease of aging.

Aging, as a stable disturbance of all three major homeostats, has to be generated by one mechanism, and this is why we can theorize that the only organ in the body, namely the hypothalamus, controls all homeostats in the organs where all changes related to aging originate. Because the hypothalamus exerts its control of homeostasis by influencing hormones, aging can be considered a hormonal disease.

Chapter 30

Two Diseases in Endocrinology

In reality, there are only two diseases in endocrinology: too much of a hormone, or too little of a hormone.

The cause of these two conditions, excess and deficiency, can be numerous, and is of utmost importance that we determine the cause. It can be physical trauma, the influence of toxins or heavy metals, hormone-producing tumors, destruction of the gland by tuberculosis, or other infections. But the treatment goal is also the same: to optimize hormone levels by treating underlying causes. Or if there is no known underlying disease, correction of hormone levels by administration of the appropriate hormone.

Signs and symptoms of hormone disorders that develop at a young age are different from those developed later in life. This is very important to distinguish because causes and treatments are different.

But as a rule, these two conditions, namely too much or too little of the hormone, display symptoms that are opposite to each other.

Too much growth hormone causes a person to grow to abnormal body height—up to 8 feet, 11 inches if the disease appears at an early age. If it starts after cessation of growth and bones are calcified, growth of cartilages and other tissues continue, and a person will have abnormally large hands and feet, chin, brow, ears, and nose, abnormally thick skin and larger than normal organs.

Too little, and you have a person of less than 4 feet, 11 inches in height with frail bones, underdeveloped muscles, elevated and unhealthy cholesterol patterns, decreased sexual capacity, depression, anxiety, fatigue, etc.

Both conditions cause shortened life spans.

If there is too much testosterone in childhood, boys achieve full sexual development by the age of 8 or younger. They are of extremely low stature due to early calcification of the bones. A beard and pubic and armpit hair appear very early in life. They have early muscle growth and body maturation and early growth of the penis and testicles. A boy appears as a very short adult at an abnormally early age, aggressive and isolated.

In girls, too much testosterone can lead to masculine body and abnormalities of the menstrual cycle, increased body hair, obesity, and infertility.

Too little testosterone in boys results in late puberty, tall stature, feminine fat pattern, underdeveloped muscles, abnormally little body hair, anemia, and passive behavior.

In the case of thyroid hormone, when there is too much of it, chemical reactions in the body go too fast. The patient is very thin, unable to gain weight (or losing weight), very nervous, hands shake, heartbeat very fast with frequent palpitations, always hot, stool too loose, unable to sleep, temperature elevated, low cholesterol and sugar, thoughts are rushing.

When there is too little, it is just the opposite: gaining weight and unable to lose it, very slow movements, slow heart rate, always cold, constipated, depressed, temperature low, cholesterol and sugar high, slow thoughts and reactions, bags under eyes.

In the case of cortisol, too much of it causes Cushing's syndrome. It presents as an accumulation of fat in the middle of the body, mostly the chest and abdomen, round red face, thick neck with a hump of the back of the neck (called "buffalo hump"), weak and thin legs, and decreased activity of the immune system. Patients with Cushing's syndrome have severely elevated blood pressure, which is almost impossible to control, and elevated blood sugar. Cushing's syndrome, if untreated, usually results in death from strokes, heart attacks, infections, or complications of diabetes.

On the other hand, too little cortisol results in Addison's disease (also known as bronze disease because of typical skin discoloration), which presents with weight loss, extremely low blood pressure and blood sugar, over-expressed inflammation and allergies, depression, and in many cases, early death due to precipitous drop in blood pressure.

There is no need to list all the hormones as a demonstration; the picture is clear—nearly every specific symptom of hormone deficiency will be the opposite of the corresponding symptom of hormone excess.

Hormone deficiencies and excesses both cause poor quality of life, development of other diseases and conditions, and lower life expectancy.

In other words, chemical processes in the body are dysregulated. Symptoms of deficiencies are opposite those of excesses. Both need to be treated in an attempt to normalize hormone levels.

The same applies to changes in hormones as a result of aging. Some hormones decline and need to be replaced, while some are produced in excess and need to be controlled. These deficiencies and excesses are just not as severe as the presence of frank endocrine diseases, but they occur in all aging people and negatively affect them. Endocrinologists, in most cases, treat severe endocrine diseases and accept age-related hormonal shifts as something natural—just because they occur in everyone.

This is why Anti-aging Functional Medicine developed into a distinct medical specialty dedicated to gently and carefully rebalancing hormonal levels, normalizing processes in a body disturbed by aging, and limiting the number of medications used to treat the results of the aging process. These medications often have adverse side effects that need to be treated by yet more medications.

Anti-aging Functional Medicine treats quality of life and optimal levels of hormones as the most important parameters of healthy aging.

Chapter 31

To Treat or Not to Treat—That Is the Question

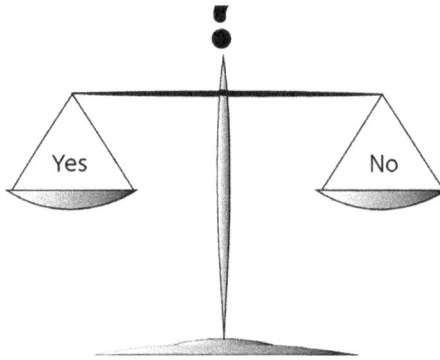

To treat or not to treat?

I n previous chapters, we briefly explained the processes of aging, or the development of the normal diseases of aging, caused by the changes in energy, adaptation, and reproduction homeostats that inevitably occur in humans if they survive past reproductive age. The longer we live, the more prominent these changes will become. The longer the average life span, the more advanced diseases of aging we will encounter.

After learning the actions of major hormones and the symptoms and signs of their deficiencies and excesses, everyone over the age of 40 who looks at the changes in hormone levels over time will see a similar pattern in themselves. In the beginning, proper diet and nutrition, behavior modification, and regular, well-designed exercise will

126

postpone the decline. Still, at some point, these healthy interventions will not be able to counteract the inevitable progression of aging.

We are facing the question of whether to treat these hormone imbalances or let nature take its course.

In the beginning, these hormonal changes do not constitute the clear endocrine diseases like diabetes, hypothyroidism, Cushing's disease, or hypogonadism as defined by reference ranges in laboratories. But medicine is not a digital discipline, and there exists the so-called "third state", which is the state between health and disease where changes are still reversible by non-aggressive interventions.

Metabolic syndrome, diabetes, hypertension, arteriosclerosis, and sarcopenia (muscle loss) do not develop overnight and do not require multiple medications with numerous side effects. Normalizing processes in the body provides an alternative way of controlling and slowing the mechanism of aging.

As every medical intervention requires a careful risk versus benefits analysis, the decision in regard to the implementation of hormone replacement therapy is between you and your doctor.

You just need to have accurate information to make your own decision as to how to approach your aging process.

There are always two points of view.

The first is that aging is inevitable, and anything beyond diet, nutritional supplements, and exercise will not be a natural, healthy approach to aging and life in general.

This approach will prolong and mitigate the aging process. However, at a certain point in life, aging takes its toll. The natural diseases of aging are progressing, and conventional medications to control the consequences will be needed to prolong life.

The other approach is to utilize all anti-aging measures based on our knowledge of the processes and shifts that are taking place in an aging organism and mitigate their effects.

Of course, proper diet, exercise, and behavior modifications conducive to anti-aging are the foundation and without them, other measures will not be effective. But without proper regulation of cellular functions, these lifestyle changes will not significantly change the progression of the general process of deterioration.

We know that levels of certain hormones decline with age: growth hormone, testosterone, DHEA, estradiol, progesterone, thyroid, and melatonin. These are hormones that contribute to the development and maintenance of the body. The other hormones, such as cortisol and insulin, even though vitally important, are major contributors to the aging process as age increases.

This is why the careful correction of hormonal levels and functions by appropriate therapies provide powerful metabolic support in slowing an aging process and helping to maintain a higher level of physical and mental activity.

Our goal in anti-aging therapy is to decrease the hormones that increase due to the aging process, namely insulin and cortisol, and supplement the body with hormones that decline in the natural process of aging.

Avoidance of fast-acting carbohydrates and sugars and physical exercise together with supplementation necessary to improve the function of insulin receptors will decrease the levels of insulin and improve insulin sensitivity.

Mental hygiene, stress management, meditation, yoga, tai chi or qigong, use of guided imagery for stress reduction, and a healthy level of exercise that does not overwhelm the adaptation system will lower the level of cortisol and mitigate the state of increased stress, hyperadaptosis.

Halting alcohol and tobacco use will improve sexual function for a while.

But at a certain age, low levels of sex hormones will reach a point when sexual activity ceases. Symptoms of sex hormone deficiencies can be controlled by herbs and supplements only if ovaries and testicles retain some degree of functional integrity, but not beyond.

Calorie restriction can prevent weight gain due to thyroid hypofunction for only so long before malnourishment becomes a problem.

At a certain point, in order to live a full-spectrum life, hormone therapy becomes a necessity.

At the same time, implementation of hormone replacement therapy does not diminish the value of nutrition, exercise, and mental balance—on the contrary, it amplifies their effectiveness.

Gradual decline in physical, sexual, and mental status can be effectively slowed down, and in many cases improved, utilizing a balanced program of nutritional management, physical exercise, and hormone replacement therapies.

It is necessary to take into consideration that, unfortunately, it is not a common medical practice to check hormone levels at the height of the reproductive period, or between 25 and 30 years of age. This would be very helpful in estimating and planning hormone replacement in later years. But what should be considered healthy hormone levels?

Usually, when we look at most laboratory test results, next to our level, we see what we call normal ranges. These are not really the "normal" ranges, but instead are reference ranges—these are not the same thing.

Here is an example. "Normal" range for height in 19-year-old men is between 5 feet, 4 inches and 6 feet, 3 inches. Nobody would disagree that the 5-foot-4 man is very short, and the 6-foot-3 man is very tall, but both are considered normal.

When establishing reference ranges for a test, laboratories perform this test on a significant number of healthy people. People are considered "healthy" if they do not have a diagnosis that may affect this particular parameter. After that, the bell curve is plotted, and two statistical deviations of 5% are cut off from both ends. This is the reference range: from the 5th percentile to the 95th percentile. The same is applied to hormone levels. For testosterone levels, the reference range is 245 to 850, but testosterone of 250 is very low for a normal 35-year-old man.

He will not look exactly like a eunuch, but his testosterone levels would correspond to a man with one testicle removed.

The other factor that needs to be considered is that we do not measure the action of hormones on the cells. As I described in previous chapters, this action is dependent on many factors—presence or absence of receptors, the status of receptors, the activity and presence of second messengers, the status of intracellular transporters. The only thing we measure is the amount of hormone in a unit of volume. This is also affected by the tissue that we test.

In the case of blood, we test the concentration of a hormone at the moment of blood collection, and as you know by now, these concentrations are changing every minute. Imagine if you are testing blood cortisol levels in a person who was running late to her laboratory appointment and was stuck in traffic—or someone who is going to court for a divorce hearing right after the blood test. Cortisol level will be greatly elevated.

In the case of 24-hour urine collection, we measure how much of a hormone is made during a 24-hour period. In this case, the levels of testosterone will be affected by the sexual or physical activity of a person throughout the 24 hours.

When we measure hormones in the saliva, levels would be affected by the status of salivary glands.

The best approach to interpreting test results is to correlate them with clinical signs and symptoms of hormone imbalances.

For example, a person with signs of thyroid insufficiency, low normal levels of thyroid hormones, and a high-normal level of thyroid stimulating hormone (TSH), does have clinically low thyroid function even though levels are not outside the reference range.

When talking about reliance on laboratory testing, an old joke comes to mind. When caught in bed with another man, the wife asks her husband, "Who are you going to believe, me or your lying eyes?"

The goal of functional medicine is to bring hormones to an optimal range which is usually close to levels of a 30-year-old person.

Of course, it is important to take into consideration that before initiating hormone replacement therapy, it is mandatory to rule out many conditions that may present themselves as (or be a cause of) hormone imbalances. For example, fatigue, which is a symptom of many hormone deficiencies, can also be the first symptom of almost any disease or condition—cancer, diabetes, and depression, to name a few. The other important aspect is to make sure that there are no contraindications to hormone replacement therapy. This is where the expertise of an experienced physician is invaluable.

Chapter 32

Hormonophobia

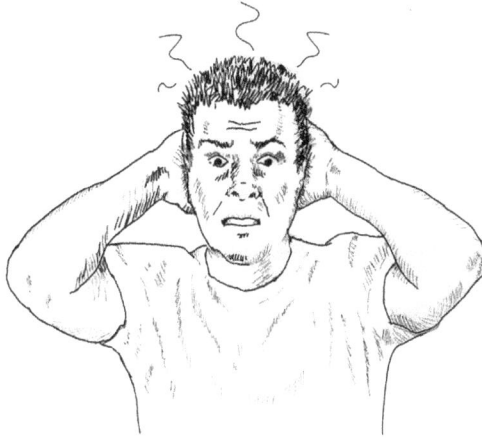

The World Health Organization defines health as "A state of complete physical, mental and social well-being and not merely the absence of disease or infirmity." Isn't it the goal of any doctor to return their patients to this state of health as defined by WHO?

Now let us look at a 60-year-old patient who does not have any disease or infirmity, whose diagnostic tests are negative and laboratory values within the reference range.

Of course, many at this age are youthful, have no "conditions," and are not taking any medications—but they are not the majority.

Most people 60 and over in the United States take some kind of medication. It may be cholesterol medicine or a blood pressure pill, or maybe diabetic medication or antacid.

Most of them will talk of the years past as the best time of their life, when they felt young, active, had a good sex drive, and were active. They sigh, remembering that feeling, and complain that they are past their peak. They obviously do not fall under the definition of health as defined by WHO.

And most of them still have a long road ahead because the average life expectancy in the US is now around 76 years and many people live past 80 years of age.

However, many doctors suffer from *hormonophobia*, a term that was coined by Dr. Cadegiani, an endocrinologist from Brazil.

Phobia is an "extreme or irrational fear of or aversion to something," as defined by the New Oxford American Dictionary.

Dr. Cadegiani defined hormonophobia as fear, detestation, dread, frightened feelings related to the most remote possibility of hormone use in a non-absolutely-severe hormone insufficiency (even with clear clinical indication and multiple benefits).

In these doctors' views, once a patient starts hormone therapy at any dose and even for a short time, all other risks for any type of disease become non-existent, and any complication or disease is automatically attributed to the use of hormones—even if this effect of hormone therapy has never been described in the medical literature before and even if the patient had risk factors in the past.

Any case report, even unrelated to hormone use, will mandatorily be linked to the use of a hormone even if the incidence of this risk factor is lower than in the general population. Any eventual possibility of any risk nullifies the clinical use of certain hormones.

The patient's response to the treatment, his desires, and his quality of life are not taken into consideration.

This type of clinical thinking does not happen with other types of medication.

Hormonophobia even goes as far as a doctor's fear and resistance to studying medical literature about the advantages and risks of the use of hormones and coming to their own conclusions.

Common hormone therapies that are accepted by hormonophobic doctors are the ones that the conventional medical community considers safe even if they are prescribed to cause disease. Take the case of birth control pills that disrupt normal ovulation and literally create a disease of infertility in young women.

A hormonophobic doctor will always mention heart attack or cancer as a reason to disavow hormone therapy. Breast cancer in the case of female HRT and prostate cancer in the case of male testosterone replacement—or just cancer if talking about growth hormone.

The multiple positive effects of hormone therapies are usually ignored and forgotten.

The only hormones that hormonophobic doctors use are the ones that are patented and promoted by pharmaceutical companies.

Take the case of the Women's Health Initiative (WHI) study. This study was stopped early due to the increased incidence of heart attack, strokes, and breast cancer in the subject population. It was immediately attributed to hormone replacement therapy.

In this study, women received treatment with Premarin, which is an estrogen extracted from pregnant mares, and Provera, an artificially altered progesterone molecule. These medications are not identical to the estradiol and progesterone produced in human females. Hormones were also taken in pill form—not delivered in the blood (bypassing the liver), the natural way of hormone metabolism. Despite these issues, the North American Menopause Society declared hormone replacement therapy dangerous.

But after several years and more analysis of data from the Women's Health Initiative study, it was concluded that even horse estrogen, taken without the artificial progesterone Provera, resulted in a lower incidence of breast cancer than in women who were not on hormone therapy at all.

Hormonophobia not only affects doctors. It also is prevalent, though becoming less and less, in patients.

How many times do hormone doctors need to remind concerned patients that breast cancer is not the only cause of death in females?

Twenty percent of people who sustained a fracture of the neck of the femur die within one year after the event, and hormone decline is the major cause of bone fragility in the elderly.

How many women and men die from conditions brought about by metabolic syndrome, which is slowed down or prevented by hormone therapies?

But death is not the worst-case scenario—prolonged suffering and loss of quality of life are.

How many patients are treated with multiple medications, one for each symptom of hormone deficiency?

Many hormone deficiencies have mild depression as a symptom. Prescribed treatment: antidepressant.

Progesterone deficiency in PMS and menopause, and testosterone deficiency in men cause insomnia. Prescribed: sleeping pill.

High blood pressure as a result of stress and overproduction of cortisol. Prescribed: blood pressure pill.

A typical elderly patient is taking the following medications.

One to lower cholesterol, one or two for blood pressure, an anti-inflammatory pill for arthritis and muscle aches, an antacid for heartburns, a sleeping pill. The hormonophobic doctor clearly does not have a side-effect phobia.

Have you ever seen TV ads promoting anti-rheumatoid medications? Autoimmune disorders are common in the elderly and are one of the normal diseases of aging. Did you listen to the list of side effects for these wonder drugs?

Of course, hormone replacement therapies also have their risks, and they are not to be discarded, but they are taken into consideration and minimized by an experienced hormone replacement physician.

But in the case of a physician who suffers from hormonophobia, natural physiologic substances which are still circulating in your body (although in insufficient amounts) are considered dangerous drugs, and supplementing hormones is equal to quackery—even though hormone replacement therapy, according to medical literature, is one of the safest medical interventions known.

In Conclusion

This book is not written to give instructions on how to prolong life or avoid aging. Nor is it a manual on hormone replacement therapy or treatment of endocrine abnormalities.

I endeavored to describe complicated processes that occur in the body with advancing age from birth to death, and mechanisms of the aging process in simple terms for readers who are interested in this subject.

As average life expectancy is increasing, it is important to prolong the active, productive, and joyful part of it, and minimize the period of debility, dependency, and dementia.

Stanislav Belkovsky, a Russian political analyst and philosopher states that old age is a psychological phenomenon. In his view, life is divided into two parts, formation and maturity, and that even in advanced age, people can be astute, productive, and active.

I am convinced that an understanding of the process of aging in some detail will give my reader some ideas of how to slow it down.

Armed with the knowledge acquired from this book about nine diseases of aging, the reader may start paying more attention to the early warning signs and take preemptive action that may postpone or even halt their development.

As human beings, we instinctively resist orders and directions when we do not clearly understand their goal and logic, but we will follow them carefully when it has been clearly explained why our life depends on following them.

This is why I have hope that this book will make a difference in improving the quality of life of all those who read it.

Bibliography

Dilman V.M. The Grand Biological Clock
English translation, Mir Publishers, 1989
ISBN 5-03-000769-5

1. Agirbasli M, Tanrikulu AM, Berenson GS. GS. Metabolic Syndrome: Bridging the Gap from Childhood to Adulthood. Cardiovasc Ther. 2016 Feb;34(1):30-6. doi: 10.1111/1755-5922.12165. Review. PubMed [citation] PMID: 26588351

2. Ambrosi TH, Scialdone A, Graja A, Gohlke S, Jank AM, Bocian C, Woelk L, Fan H, Logan DW, Schürmann A, Saraiva LR, Schulz TJ. Adipocyte Accumulation in the Bone Marrow during Obesity and Aging Impairs Stem Cell-Based Hematopoietic and Bone Regeneration. Cell Stem Cell. 2017 Jun 1;20(6):771-784.e6. doi: 10.1016/j.stem.2017.02.009. Epub 2017 Mar 16. PubMed [citation] PMID: 28330582, PMCID: PMC5459794

3. Andersen ME, Barton HA. Biological regulation of receptor-hormone complex concentrations in relation to dose-response assessments for endocrine-active compounds. Toxicol Sci. 1999 Mar;48(1):38-50. Review. PubMed [citation] PMID: 10330682

4. Appelman-Dijkstra NM, Claessen KM, Roelfsema F, Pereira AM, Biermasz NR. Long-term effects of recombinant human GH replacement in adults with GH deficiency: a systematic review. Eur J Endocrinol. 2013

May 28;169(1):R1-14. doi: 10.1530/EJE-12-1088. Print 2013 Jul. Review. PubMed [citation] PMID: 23572082

5. Aschheim P. [Reactivation of the ovary of senile rats in permanent estrus by means of gonadotropic hormones or placement in darkness]. C R Acad Hebd Seances Acad Sci D. 1965 May 24;260(21):5627-30. French. No abstract available. PubMed [citation] PMID: 4953963

6. ASCHHEIM P. [Permanent estrus and prolactin]. C R Hebd Seances Acad Sci. 1962 Nov 26;255:3053-5. French. No abstract available. PubMed [citation] PMID: 13965130

7. ASCHHEIM P. [The effect of decidual tissue on pseudopregnancy induced by administration of prolactin in the rats]. C R Seances Soc Biol Fil. 1954 Jan;148(1-2):185-7. Undetermined Language. No abstract available. PubMed [citation] PMID: 13161409

8. ASCHHEIM P. [Repeated pseudogestation in senile rats]. C R Hebd Seances Acad Sci. 1961 Oct 30;253:1988-90. French. No abstract available. PubMed [citation] PMID: 13862764

9. ASCHHEIM P. [History of the biological diagnosis of pregnancy]. Brux Med. 1954 Nov 28;34(48):2355-62. French. No abstract available. PubMed [citation] PMID: 13209220

10. ASCHHEIM P, PASTEELS JL. [HISTOPHYSIOLOGICAL STUDY OF PROLACTIN SECRETION IN SENILE FEMALE RATS]. C R Hebd Seances Acad Sci. 1963 Aug 5;257:1373-5. French. No abstract available. PubMed [citation] PMID: 14120937

11. Aschheim P. [Hypothalamic regulation of the LH gonadotropic function in the senile rat: contribution to the study of "deficient cells" in the ovarian interstium]. Arch Anat Histol Embryol. 1968;51(1):53-63. French. No abstract available. PubMed [citation] PMID: 4905282

12. 12. Aschheim P. [Pituitary content of luteinizing hormone (LH) and histophysiologic reaction with circulating LH of ovarian interstitial tissue in different types of senial rats]. C R Acad Hebd Seances Acad Sci D. 1968 Oct 21;267(17):1397-400. French. No abstract available. PubMed [citation]

PMID: 4972972

13. *Aschheim P. A biological aging test for the central regulation of the estrous cycle in the rat. Its first application. Experientia. 1974 Feb 15;30(2):213. No abstract available. PubMed [citation] PMID: 4856011*

14. *ASCHHEIM P. [RESULTS PROVIDED BY HETEROCHRONIC GRAFTS OF THE OVARIES IN THE STUDY OF THE HYPOTHALAMO-HYPOPHYSO-OVARIAN REGULATION OF SENILE RATS]. Gerontologia. 1964-1965;10:65-75. French. No abstract available. PubMed [citation] PMID: 14312531*

15. *ASCHHEIM P, NETTER A. [Inhibitory effect of thallium on ovulation induced in the rabbit]. Ann Endocrinol (Paris). 1957 May-Jun;18(3):427-36. French. No abstract available. PubMed [citation] PMID: 13470410*

16. *ASCHHEIM S, VARANGOT J, VASSY S, ASCHHEIM P. [Positive biological pregnancy tests and false pregnancy]. Bull Fed Soc Gynecol Obstet Lang Fr. 1952;4(4):664-7. Undetermined Language. No abstract available. PubMed [citation] PMID: 13009281*

17. *Axelrod J, Reisine TD. Stress hormones: their interaction and regulation. Science. 1984 May 4;224(4648):452-9. Review. PubMed [citation] PMID: 6143403*

18. *Bain J. Testosterone and the aging male: to treat or not to treat? Maturitas.2010 May;66(1):16-22. doi: 10.1016/j.maturitas.2010.01.009. Epub 2010 Feb 13. Review. PubMed [citation] PMID: 20153946*

19. *Barbesino G. Thyroid Function Changes in the Elderly and Their Relationship to Cardiovascular Health: A Mini-Review. Gerontology. 2019;65(1):1-8. doi: 10.1159/000490911. Epub 2018 Jul 20. Review. PubMed [citation] PMID: 30032140*

20. *Bartke A, Matt KS, Steger RW, Clayton RN, Chandrashekar V, Smith MS. Role of prolactin in the regulation of sensitivity of the hypothalamic-pituitary system to steroid feedback. Adv Exp Med Biol. 1987;219:153-75. Review. PubMed [citation] PMID: 3324676*

21. *Bell FR. Hypothalamic control of food intake. Proc Nutr Soc. 1971 Sep;30(2):103-9. Review. No abstract available. PubMed [citation] PMID:*

22. Bentley RA, Ross CN, O'Brien MJ. Obesity, Metabolism, and Aging: A Multiscalar Approach. Prog Mol Biol Transl Sci. 2018;155:25-42. doi: 10.1016/bs.pmbts.2017.11.016. Epub 2018 Feb 1. Review. PubMed [citation] PMID: 29653680

23. Berczi I. Pituitary hormones and immune function. Acta Paediatr Suppl. 1997 Nov;423:70-5. Review. PubMed [citation] PMID: 9401545

24. Berenson GS; Bogalusa Heart Study group.. Health consequences of obesity. Pediatr Blood Cancer. 2012 Jan;58(1):117-21. doi: 10.1002/pbc.23373. PubMed [citation] PMID: 22076834

25. Bierman EL, Porte D Jr. Carbohydrate intolerance and lipemia. Ann Intern Med. 1968 Apr;68(4):926-33. Review. No abstract available. PubMed [citation] PMID: 4870575

26. 26. Bierman EL, Nelson R. Carbohydrates, diabetes, and blood lipids. World Rev Nutr Diet. 1975;22:280-7. Review. No abstract available. PubMed [citation] PMID: 1103486

27. Bierman EL. Fat metabolism, atherosclerosis and aging in man: a review. Mech Ageing Dev. 1973 Oct-Nov;2(4):315-32. Review. No abstract available. PubMed [citation] PMID: 4591681

28. Bischof GN, Park DC. Obesity and Aging: Consequences for Cognition, Brain Structure, and Brain Function. Psychosom Med. 2015 Jul-Aug;77(6):697-709. doi: 10.1097/PSY.0000000000000212. Review. PubMed [citation] PMID: 26107577, PMCID: PMC5648343

29. Blackman MR. Pituitary hormones and aging. Endocrinol Metab Clin North Am. 1987 Dec;16(4):981-94. Review. PubMed [citation] PMID: 2828042

30. Bourguignon JP, Gerard A, Mathieu J, Mathieu A, Franchimont P. Maturation of the hypothalamic control of pulsatile gonadotropin-releasing hormone secretion at onset of puberty. I. Increased activation of N-methyl-D-aspartate receptors.Endocrinology. 1990 Aug;127(2):873-81. PubMed [citation] PMID: 2164923

31. *Boyar RM. Sleep-related endocrine rhythms. Res Publ Assoc Res Nerv Ment Dis. 1978;56:373-86. No abstract available. PubMed [citation] PMID: 23575*

32. *Carlson HE, Hershman JM. The hypothalamic-pituitary-thyroid axis. Med Clin North Am. 1975 Sep;59(5):1045-53. Review. PubMed [citation] PMID: 808671*

33. *COURRIER R, GUILLEMINR, JUTISZ M, SAKIZ E, ASCHHEIM P. [Presence in an extract of hypothalamus of a substance stimulating the secretion of the luteinizing hormone of the anterior pituitary (LH)]. C R Hebd Seances Acad Sci. 1961 Aug 7;253:922-7. French. No abstract available. PubMed [citation] PMID: 13881740*

34. *Crews D. Evolution of neuroendocrine mechanisms that regulate sexual behavior. Trends Endocrinol Metab. 2005 Oct;16(8):354-61. Review. PubMed [citation] PMID: 16139506*

35. *Crumeyrolle-Arias M, Scheib D, Aschheim P. Light and electron microscopy of the ovarian interstitial tissue in the senile rat: normal aspect and response to HCG of 'deficiency cells' and 'epithelial cords'. Gerontology. 1976;22(3):185-204. PubMed [citation] PMID: 1261809*

36. *Crumeyrolle-Arias M, Aschheim P. Post-hypophysectomy ovarian senescence and its relation to the spontaneous structural changes in the ovary of intact aged rats. Gerontology. 1981;27(1-2):58-71. PubMed [citation] PMID: 7215821*

37. *Crumeyrolle-Arias M, Aschheim P. [Secretion of ovarian estrogen induced by HCG in immature hypophysectomised rats]. C R Acad Hebd Seances Acad Sci D. 1976 Jun 28;282(24):2207-10. French. PubMed [citation] PMID: 822956*

38. *Curtò L, Trimarchi F. Hypopituitarism in the elderly: a narrative review on clinical management of hypothalamic-pituitary-gonadal, hypothalamic-pituitary-thyroid and hypothalamic-pituitary-adrenal axes dysfunction. J Endocrinol Invest. 2016 Oct;39(10):1115-24. doi: 10.1007/s40618-016-0487-8. Epub 2016 May 21. Review. PubMed [citation] PMID: 27209187*

39. *Davis PJ. Ageing and endocrine function. Clin Endocrinol Metab. 1979*

Nov;8(3):603-19. Review. No abstract available. PubMed [citation] PMID: 389493

40. *De Kloet ER, Sutanto W, Rots N, van Haarst A, van den Berg D, Oitzl M, van Eekelen A, Voorhuis D. Plasticity and function of brain corticosteroid receptors during aging. Acta Endocrinol (Copenh). 1991;125 Suppl 1:65-72. Review. PubMed [citation] PMID: 1801504*

41. *De Libero G, Mori L. How T lymphocytes recognize lipid antigens. FEBS Lett. 2006 Oct 9;580(23):5580-7. Epub 2006 Aug 28. Review. PubMed [citation] PMID: 16949584*

42. *Diamanti-Kandarakis E, Dattilo M, Macut D, Duntas L, Gonos ES, Goulis DG, Gantenbein CK, Kapetanou M, Koukkou E, Lambrinoudaki I, Michalaki M, Eftekhari-Nader S, Pasquali R, Peppa M, Tzanela M, Vassilatou E, Vryonidou A; COMBO ENDO TEAM: 2016.. MECHANISMS IN ENDOCRINOLOGY: Aging and anti-aging: a Combo-Endocrinology overview. Eur J Endocrinol. 2017 Jun;176(6):R283-R308. doi: 10.1530/ EJE-16-1061. Epub 2017 Mar 6. Review. PubMed [citation] PMID: 28264815*

43. *Dilman VM. Age-associated elevation of hypothalamic, threshold to feedback control, and its role in development, ageing, and disease. Lancet. 1971 Jun 12;1(7711):1211-9. No abstract available. PubMed [citation] PMID: 4103080*

44. *DOLE VP, GORDIS E, BIERMAN EL. HYPERLIPEMIA AND ARTERIOSCLEROSIS. N Engl J Med. 1963 Sep 26;269:686-9. Review. No abstract available. PubMed [citation] PMID: 14050974*

45. *Duntas LH. Thyroid Function in Aging: A Discerning Approach. Rejuvenation Res. 2018 Feb;21(1):22-28. doi: 10.1089/rej.2017.1991. Epub 2017 Aug 28. Review. PubMed [citation] PMID: 28661207*

46. *Fayein NA, Aschheim P. Age-related temporal changes of levels of circulating progesterone in repeatedly pseudopregnant rats. Biol Reprod. 1980Oct;23(3):616-20. No abstract available. PubMed [citation] PMID: 7448264*

47. *Ferrari E, Casarotti D, Muzzoni B, Albertelli N, Cravello L, Fioravanti*

M, Solerte SB, Magri F. *Age-related changes of the adrenal secretory pattern: possible role in pathological brain aging. Brain Res Brain Res Rev. 2001 Nov;37(1-3):294-300. Review. PubMed [citation] PMID: 11744094*

48. *Gáliková M, Klepsatel P. Obesity and Aging in the Drosophila Model. Int J Mol Sci. 2018 Jun 27;19(7). pii: E1896. doi: 10.3390/ijms19071896. Review. PubMed [citation] PMID: 29954158, PMCID: PMC6073435*

49. *Garcia-Segura LM, Veiga S, Sierra A, Melcangi RC, Azcoitia I. Aromatase: a neuroprotective enzyme. Prog Neurobiol. 2003 Sep;71(1):31-41. Review. PubMed [citation] PMID: 14611865*

50. *Gauthier BR, Sola-García A, Cáliz-Molina MÁ, Lorenzo PI, Cobo-Vuilleumier N, Capilla-González V, Martin-Montalvo A. Thyroid hormones in diabetes, cancer, and aging. Aging Cell. 2020 Nov;19(11):e13260. doi: 10.1111/acel.13260. Epub 2020 Oct 13. Review. PubMed [citation] PMID: 33048427, PMCID: PMC7681062*

51. *Giordano R, Aimaretti G, Lanfranco F, Bo M, Baldi M, Broglio F, Baldelli R, Grottoli S, Ghigo E, Arvat E. Testing pituitary function in aging individuals.Endocrinol Metab Clin North Am. 2005 Dec;34(4):895-906, viii-ix. Review. No abstract available. PubMed [citation] PMID: 16310629*

52. *Gompel A. Progesterone, progestins and the endometrium in perimenopause and in menopausal hormone therapy. Climacteric. 2018 Aug;21(4):321-325. doi: 10.1080/13697137.2018.1446932. Epub 2018 Mar 27. Review. PubMed [citation] PMID: 29583028*

53. *Goya RG, Brown OA, Bolognani F. The thymus-pituitary axis and its changes during aging. Neuroimmunomodulation. 1999 Jan-Apr;6(1-2):137-42. Review. PubMed [citation] PMID: 9876244*

54. *Guay AT. Testosterone and erectile physiology. Aging Male. 2006 Dec;9(4):201-6. Review. PubMed [citation] PMID: 17178555*

55. *Gupta D, Morley JE. Hypothalamic-pituitary-adrenal (HPA) axis and aging. Compr Physiol. 2014 Oct;4(4):1495-510. doi: 10.1002/cphy. c130049. Review. PubMed [citation] PMID: 25428852*

56. *Gupta D. Hypothalamic control of the mammalian sexual maturation. Padiatr Padol Suppl. 1977;(5):83-102. PubMed [citation] PMID: 335339*

57. *Hall JE, Gill S. Neuroendocrine aspects of aging in women. Endocrinol Metab Clin North Am. 2001 Sep;30(3):631-46. Review. PubMed [citation] PMID: 11571934*

58. *Harrington J, Lee-Chiong T. Obesity and aging. Clin Chest Med. 2009 Sep;30(3):609-14, x. doi: 10.1016/j.ccm.2009.05.011. Review. PubMed [citation] PMID: 19700056*

59. *Hemminki E, Topo P, Malin M, Kangas I. Physicians' views on hormone therapy around and after menopause. Maturitas. 1993 May;16(3):163-73. PubMed [citation] PMID: 8515716*

60. *Herbison AE. Control of puberty onset and fertility by gonadotropin-releasing hormone neurons. Nat Rev Endocrinol. 2016 Aug;12(8):452-66. doi: 10.1038/nrendo.2016.70. Epub 2016 May 20. Review. PubMed [citation] PMID: 27199290*

61. *Herman JP, McKlveen JM, Ghosal S, Kopp B, Wulsin A, Makinson R, Scheimann J, Myers B. Regulation of the Hypothalamic-Pituitary-Adrenocortical Stress Response. Compr Physiol. 2016 Mar 15;6(2):603-21. doi: 10.1002/cphy.c150015. Review. PubMed [citation] PMID: 27065163, PMCID: PMC4867107*

62. *Hirsch H. Facing Provider Misconceptions Towards the Use of Hormone Therapy in 2020. J Gen Intern Med. 2021 Mar;36(3):767-768. doi: 10.1007/s11606-020-05940-w. Epub 2020 Jun 4. No abstract available. PubMed [citation] PMID: 32500331, PMCID: PMC7947121*

63. *Holtorf K. The bioidentical hormone debate: are bioidentical hormones (estradiol, estriol, and progesterone) safer or more efficacious than commonly used synthetic versions in hormone replacement therapy? Postgrad Med. 2009 Jan;121(1):73-85. doi: 10.3810/pgm.2009.01.1949. Review. PubMed [citation] PMID: 19179815*

64. *Horvath TL, Garcia-Segura LM, Naftolin F. Control of gonadotropin feedback: the possible role of estrogen-induced hypothalamic synaptic plasticity. Gynecol Endocrinol. 1997 Apr;11(2):139-43. Review. PubMed [citation] PMID: 9174856*

65. *Hua JT, Hildreth KL, Pelak VS. Effects of Testosterone Therapy on*

Cognitive Function in Aging: A Systematic Review. Cogn Behav Neurol. 2016 Sep;29(3):122-38. doi: 10.1097/WNN.0000000000000104. Review. PubMed [citation] PMID: 27662450, PMCID: PMC5079177

66. *Hunte C, Richers S. Lipids and membrane protein structures. Curr Opin Struct Biol. 2008 Aug;18(4):406-11. doi: 10.1016/j.sbi.2008.03.008. Epub 2008 May 19. Review. PubMed [citation] PMID: 18495472*

67. *Ibayashi H, Kato K, Motomatsu T, Nawada H, Wasada T. [Senescence and hormones]. Nihon Rinsho. 1974 Jan;32(1):20-9. Review. Japanese. No abstract available. PubMed [citation] PMID: 4364038*

68. *Jacobson L, Sapolsky R. The role of the hippocampus in feedback regulation of the hypothalamic-pituitary-adrenocortical axis. Endocr Rev. 1991 May;12(2):118-34. Review. PubMed [citation] PMID: 2070776*

69. *Jafurulla M, Chattopadhyay A. Membrane lipids in the function of serotonin and adrenergic receptors. Curr Med Chem. 2013;20(1):47-55. Review. PubMed [citation] PMID: 23151002*

70. *Jasim S, Gharib H. THYROID AND AGING. Endocr Pract. 2018 Apr;24(4):369-374. doi: 10.4158/EP171796.RA. Epub 2017 Aug 17. Review. PubMed [citation] PMID: 28816538*

71. *Jones CM, Boelaert K. The Endocrinology of Ageing: A Mini-Review. Gerontology. 2015;61(4):291-300. doi: 10.1159/000367692. Epub 2014 Nov 27. Review. PubMed [citation] PMID: 25471682*

72. *Juonala M, Magnussen CG, Berenson GS, Venn A, Burns TL, Sabin MA, Srinivasan SR, Daniels SR, Davis PH, Chen W, Sun C, Cheung M, Viikari JS, Dwyer T, Raitakari OT. Childhood adiposity, adult adiposity, and cardiovascular risk factors. N Engl J Med. 2011 Nov 17;365(20):1876-85. doi: 10.1056/NEJMoa1010112. PubMed [citation] PMID: 22087679*

73. *Kaplan B, Rabinerson D, Yogev Y, Bar-Hava I, Bar J, Orvieto R. A survey of physicians' attitude and approach to hormone replacement therapy during\ menopuase. Clin Exp Obstet Gynecol. 2002;29(1):31-3. PubMed [citation] PMID: 12013088*

74. *Keller-Wood ME, Dallman MF. Corticosteroid inhibition of ACTH secretion. Endocr Rev. 1984 Winter;5(1):1-24. Review. PubMed [citation]*

PMID: 6323158

75. *Kenemans P, van Unnik GA, Mijatovic V, van der Mooren MJ. Perspectives in hormone replacement therapy. Maturitas. 2001 Jun 15;38 Suppl 1:S41-8. Review. PubMed [citation] PMID: 11390123*

76. *Khlebnikov VV, Kuznetsov SL, Chernov DA, Agrytskov AM, Ahmad A, Nor-Ashikin MN, Ullah M, Kapitonova MY. [Age-related peculiarities of thehypothalamo-hypophyseo-adrenal system in chronic heterotypic stress]. Morfologiia. 2015;147(1):15-20. Russian. PubMed [citation] PMID: 25958723*

77. *Kim JK, Alley D, Hu P, Karlamangla A, Seeman T, Crimmins EM. Changes in postmenopausal hormone therapy use since 1988. Womens Health Issues. 2007 Nov-Dec;17(6):338-41. Epub 2007 Oct 22. Review. No abstract available. PubMed [citation] PMID: 17936641, PMCID: PMC2180400*

78. *Kinsella JE. Lipids, membrane receptors, and enzymes: effects of dietary fatty acids. JPEN J Parenter Enteral Nutr. 1990 Sep-Oct;14(5 Suppl):200S-217S. Review. PubMed [citation] PMID: 2232105*

79. *Kolip P, Hoefling-Engels N, Schmacke N. Attitudes toward postmenopausal long-term hormone therapy. Qual Health Res. 2009 Feb;19(2):207-15. doi: 10.1177/1049732308328053. Epub 2008 Dec 2. PubMed [citation] PMID: 19050178*

80. *Lage R, Fernø J, Nogueiras R, Diéguez C, López M. Contribution of adaptive thermogenesis to the hypothalamic regulation of energy balance. Biochem J. 2016 Nov 15;473(22):4063-4082. Review. PubMed [citation] PMID: 27834738*

81. *Lilly MP, Gann DS. The hypothalamic-pituitary-adrenal-immune axis. A critical assessment. Arch Surg. 1992 Dec;127(12):1463-74. Review. PubMed [citation] PMID: 1365694*

82. *Lindh-Astrand L, Brynhildsen J, Hoffmann M, Liffner S, Hammar M. Attitudes towards the menopause and hormone therapy over the turn of the century. Maturitas. 2007 Jan 20;56(1):12-20. Epub 2006 Jun 23. PubMed [citation] PMID: 16797891*

83. *Little AG. A review of the peripheral levels of regulation by thyroid* *hormone. J Comp Physiol B. 2016 Aug;186(6):677-88. doi: 10.1007/s00360-016-0984-2. Epub 2016 Apr 9. Review. PubMed [citation] PMID: 27062031*

84. *Livadas S, Chrousos GP. Control of the onset of puberty. Curr Opin Pediatr. 2016 Aug;28(4):551-8. doi: 10.1097/MOP.0000000000000386. Review. PubMed [citation] PMID: 27386974*

85. *Maclean DB, Jackson IM. Molecular biology and regulation of the hypothalamic hormones. Baillieres Clin Endocrinol Metab. 1988 Nov;2(4):835-68. Review. PubMed [citation] PMID: 2908317*

86. *Mariotti S, Chiovato L, Franceschi C, Pinchera A. Thyroid autoimmunity and aging. Exp Gerontol. 1998 Sep;33(6):535-41. Review. PubMed [citation] PMID: 9789731*

87. *Mayo W, George O, Darbra S, Bouyer JJ, Vallée M, Darnaudéry M, Pallarès M, Lemaire-Mayo V, Le Moal M, Piazza PV, Abrous N. Individual differences in cognitive aging: implication of pregnenolone sulfate. Prog Neurobiol. 2003 Sep;71(1):43-8. Review. PubMed [citation] PMID: 14611866*

88. *Meade CJ, Mertin J. Fatty acids and immunity. Adv Lipid Res. 1978;16:127-65. Review. No abstract available. PubMed [citation] PMID: 362864*

89. *Miner MM, Perelman MA. A psychological perspective on male rejuvenation. Fertil Steril. 2013 Jun;99(7):1803-6. doi: 10.1016/j.fertnstert.2013.04.044. Review. PubMed [citation] PMID: 23726253*

90. *Moreau KL, Babcock MC, Hildreth KL. Sex differences in vascular aging in response to testosterone. Biol Sex Differ. 2020 Apr 15;11(1):18. doi: 10.1186/s13293-020-00294-8. Review. PubMed [citation] PMID: 32295637, PMCID: PMC7161199*

91. *Morley JE. Androgens and aging. Maturitas. 2001 Feb 28;38(1):61-71; discussion 71-3. Review. PubMed [citation] PMID: 11311591*

92. *Morley JE. Scientific overview of hormone treatment used for rejuvenation. Fertil Steril. 2013 Jun;99(7):1807-13. doi: 10.1016/j.fertnstert.2013.04.009. Review. PubMed [citation] PMID: 23726254*

93. Münzberg H, Qualls-Creekmore E, Berthoud HR, Morrison CD, Yu S. *Neural Control of Energy Expenditure. Handb Exp Pharmacol. 2016;233:173-94. doi: 10.1007/164_2015_33. Review. PubMed [citation] PMID: 26578523, PMCID: PMC4818114*

94. Nazian SJ, Mahesh VB. *Hypothalamic, pituitary, testicular, and secondary organ functions and interactions during the sexual maturation of the male rat. Arch Androl. 1980 Jun;4(4):283-303. Review. PubMed [citation] PMID: 6774676*

95. Nelson JF, Bergman MD, Karelus K, Felicio LS. *Aging of the hypothalamo-pituitary-ovarian axis: hormonal influences and cellular mechanisms. J Steroid Biochem. 1987;27(4-6):699-705. Review. PubMed [citation] PMID: 3320554*

96. NETTER A, LAMBERT A, ASCHHEIM P. *[Studies on luteal insufficiency; treatment of certain of its forms with cortisone]. Gynecol Obstet (Paris). 1955;54(5):574-84. French. No abstract available. PubMed [citation] PMID: 13305939*

97. NETTER A, HENRY R, LAMBERT A, THEVENET M, LUMBROSO P, ASCHHEIM P. *Studies on certain aspects of hyperandrogenism in women; hyperandrogenism and spaniomenorrhea; hyperandrogenism and luteal insufficiency; experiments on ovarian secretion of female androgens. Ann Endocrinol (Paris). 1955;16(6):833-48. French. No abstract available. PubMed [citation] PMID: 13327441*

98. NOVELLA MA, ALLOITEAU JJ, ASCHHEIM P. *[IS THE RAT PREPARED ACCORDING TO PARLOW'S TECHNIC SUITABLE FOR THE STUDY OF A SUBSTANCE STIMULATING DISCHARGE OF LUTEINIZING HORMONE BY THE PITUITARY?]. C R Hebd Seances Acad Sci. 1964 Aug 24;259:1553-6. French. No abstract available. PubMed [citation] PMID: 14191206*

99. Novella MA, Acker G, Alloiteau JJ, Aschheim P. *[Value of a pretreatment by a tranquilizing agent (trifluoperazine) for determination of the luteinizing hormone by Parlow's method]. C R Acad Hebd Seances Acad Sci D. 1965 Aug 18;261(7):1742-5. French. No abstract available. PubMed [citation] PMID: 4954433*

100. *Otton R, Soriano FG, Verlengia R, Curi R. Diabetes induces apoptosis in lymphocytes. J Endocrinol. 2004 Jul;182(1):145-56. PubMed [citation] PMID: 15225139*

101. *Pang ZP, Han W. Regulation of synaptic functions in central nervous system by endocrine hormones and the maintenance of energy homoeostasis. Biosci Rep. 2012 Oct;32(5):423-32. doi: 10.1042/BSR20120026. Review. PubMed [citation] PMID: 22582733, PMCID: PMC3804927*

102. *Peng MT, Huang HH. Aging of hypothalamic-pituitary-ovarian function in the rat. Fertil Steril. 1972 Aug;23(8):535-42. No abstract available. PubMed [citation] PMID: 5065232*

103. *Penning TM. Hydroxysteroid dehydrogenases and pre-receptor regulation of steroid hormone action. Hum Reprod Update. 2003 May-Jun;9(3):193-205. Review. PubMed [citation] PMID: 12861966*

104. *Pfaus JG, Kippin TE, Centeno S. Conditioning and sexual behavior: a review. Horm Behav. 2001 Sep;40(2):291-321. Review. PubMed [citation] PMID: 11534994*

105. *Piva F, Zanisi M, Motta M, Martini L. "Ultrashort" control of hypothalamic hormones secretion: a brief history. J Endocrinol Invest. 2004;27(6 Suppl):68-72. Review. PubMed [citation] PMID: 15481806*

106. *Plotsky PM, Thrivikraman KV, Meaney MJ. Central and feedback regulation of hypothalamic corticotropin-releasing factor secretion. Ciba Found Symp. 1993;172:59-75; discussion 75-84. Review. PubMed [citation] PMID: 8491095*

107. *Power ML, Zinberg S, Schulkin J. A survey of obstetrician-gynecologists concerning practice patterns and attitudes toward hormone therapy. Menopause. 2006 May-Jun;13(3):434-41. PubMed [citation] PMID: 16735940*

108. *Rakov H, De Angelis M, Renko K, Hönes GS, Zwanziger D, Moeller LC, Schramm KW, Führer D. Aging Is Associated with Low Thyroid State and Organ-Specific Sensitivity to Thyroxine. Thyroid. 2019 Dec;29(12):1723-1733. doi: 10.1089/thy.2018.0377. Epub 2019 Sep 26. PubMed [citation] PMID: 31441387*

109. *Richardson SB, Twente S. Inhibition of rat hypothalamic somatostatin release by somatostatin: evidence for somatostatin ultrashort loop feedback. Endocrinology. 1986 May;118(5):2076-82. PubMed [citation] PMID: 2870911*

110. *Roberts PJ, Sibbald B. Hormone replacement therapy: the views of general practitioners and practice nurses. Br J Gen Pract. 2000 Dec;50(461):986, 991. PubMed [citation] PMID: 11224973, PMCID: PMC1313888*

111. *Rushworth RL, Torpy DJ, Falhammar H. Adrenal crises in older patients. Lancet Diabetes Endocrinol. 2020 Jul;8(7):628-639. doi: 10.1016/ S2213-8587(20)30122-4. Review. PubMed [citation] PMID: 32559478*

112. *Sadow TF, Rubin RT. Effects of hypothalamic peptides on the aging brain. Psychoneuroendocrinology. 1992 Aug;17(4):293-314. Review. PubMed [citation] PMID: 1359604*

113. *Sahu P, Gidwani B, Dhongade HJ. Pharmacological activities of dehydroepiandrosterone: A review. Steroids. 2020 Jan;153:108507. doi: 10.1016/j.steroids.2019.108507. Epub 2019 Oct 3. Review. PubMed [citation] PMID: 31586606*

114. *114. Savine R, Sönksen PH. Is the somatopause an indication for growth hormone replacement? J Endocrinol Invest. 1999;22(5 Suppl):142-9. Review. PubMed [citation] PMID: 10442584*

115. *Schild L, Lendeckel U, Gardemann A, Wiswedel I, Schmidt CA, Wolke C, Walther R, Grabarczyk P, Busemann C. Composition of molecular cardiolipin species correlates with proliferation of lymphocytes. Exp Biol Med (Maywood). 2012 Apr;237(4):372-9. doi: 10.1258/ebm.2011.011311. Epub*

116. *Schreiber V. [Internal (short) feedback loops in the hypophyseal-hypothalamic system]. Cesk Fysiol. 1970 Sep;19(1):27-35. Review. Czech. No abstract available. PubMed [citation] PMID: 4320289*

117. *Seeman TE, Robbins RJ. Aging and hypothalamic-pituitary-adrenal response to challenge in humans. Endocr Rev. 1994 Apr;15(2):233-60. Review. No abstract available. PubMed [citation] PMID: 8026389*

118. *Seidman SN, Weiser M. Testosterone and mood in aging men. Psychiatr*

Clin North Am. 2013 Mar;36(1):177-82. doi: 10.1016/j.psc.2013.01.007. Review. PubMed [citation] PMID: 23538087 119. Smith AD, Conroy DM, Belin J. Membrane lipid modification and immune function.

119. *Proc Nutr Soc. 1985 Jul;44(2):201-9. Review. No abstract available. PubMed [citation] PMID: 3901013*

120. *Smith SM, Vale WW. The role of the hypothalamic-pituitary-adrenal axis in neuroendocrine responses to stress. Dialogues Clin Neurosci. 2006;8(4):383-95. Review. PubMed [citation] PMID: 17290797, PMCID: PMC3181830*

121. *Spector AA, Yorek MA. Membrane lipid composition and cellular function. J Lipid Res. 1985 Sep;26(9):1015-35. Review. PubMed [citation] PMID: 3906008*

122. *Stanisić V, Lonard DM, O'Malley BW. Modulation of steroid hormone receptor activity. Prog Brain Res. 2010;181:153-76. doi: 10.1016/S0079-6123(08)81009-6. Review. PubMed [citation] PMID: 20478437*

123. *Starling S. Innate lymphoid cells: Lipid surveillance by skin ILCs. Nat Rev Immunol. 2018 Feb;18(2):78-79. doi: 10.1038/nri.2018.1. Epub 2018 Jan 15. No abstract available. PubMed [citation] PMID: 29332938*

124. *Stein DG, Wright DW, Kellermann AL. Does progesterone have neuroprotective properties? Ann Emerg Med. 2008 Feb;51(2):164-72. Epub 2007 Jun 22. Review. PubMed [citation] PMID: 17588708*

125. *Sunshine H, Iruela-Arispe ML. Membrane lipids and cell signaling. Curr Opin Lipidol. 2017 Oct;28(5):408-413. doi: 10.1097/MOL.0000000000000443. Review. PubMed [citation] PMID: 28692598, PMCID: PMC5776726*

126. *Swaab DF, Bao AM, Lucassen PJ. The stress system in the human brain in depression and neurodegeneration. Ageing Res Rev. 2005 May;4(2):141-94. Review. PubMed [citation] PMID: 15996533*

127. *127. Tanaka S, Nemoto Y, Takei Y, Morikawa R, Oshima S, Nagaishi T, Okamoto R, Tsuchiya K, Nakamura T, Stutte S, Watanabe M. High-fat diet-derived free fatty acids impair the intestinal immune system and increase sensitivity to intestinal epithelial damage. Biochem Biophys Res Commun.*

2020 Feb 19;522(4):971-977. doi: 10.1016/j.bbrc.2019.11.158. Epub 2019 Dec 3. PubMed [citation] PMID: 31810607

128. *Taylor M. Alternatives to conventional hormone replacement therapy. Compr Ther. 1997 Aug;23(8):514-32. Review. PubMed [citation] PMID: 9283741*

129. *Tsitouras PD, Bulat T. The aging male reproductive system. Endocrinol Metab Clin North Am. 1995 Jun;24(2):297-315. Review. PubMed [citation] PMID: 7656893*

130. *Urban RJ. Neuroendocrinology of aging in the male and female. Endocrinol Metab Clin North Am. 1992 Dec;21(4):921-31. Review. PubMed [citation] PMID: 1486882*

131. *Vallée M, Mayo W, Le Moal M. Role of pregnenolone, dehydroepiandrosterone and their sulfate esters on learning and memory in cognitive aging. Brain Res Brain Res Rev. 2001 Nov;37(1-3):301-12. Review. PubMed [citation] PMID: 11744095*

132. *Vallée M, Purdy RH, Mayo W, Koob GF, Le Moal M. Neuroactive steroids: new biomarkers of cognitive aging. J Steroid Biochem Mol Biol. 2003 Jun;85(2-5):329-35. Review. PubMed [citation] PMID: 12943719*

133. *van den Beld AW, Kaufman JM, Zillikens MC, Lamberts SWJ, Egan JM, van der Lely AJ. The physiology of endocrine systems with ageing. Lancet Diabetes Endocrinol. 2018 Aug;6(8):647-658. doi: 10.1016/S2213-8587(18)30026-3. Epub 2018 Jul 17. Review. PubMed [citation] PMID: 30017799, PMCID: PMC6089223*

134. *Vasconsuelo A, Milanesi L, Boland R. Actions of 17β-estradiol and testosterone in the mitochondria and their implications in aging. Ageing Res Rev. 2013 Sep;12(4):907-17. doi: 10.1016/j.arr.2013.09.001. Epub 2013 Sep 14. Review. PubMed [citation] PMID: 24041489*

135. *135. Veldhuis JD, Keenan DM, Liu PY, Iranmanesh A, Takahashi PY, Nehra AX. The aging male hypothalamic-pituitary-gonadal axis: pulsatility and feedback. Mol Cell Endocrinol. 2009 Feb 5;299(1):14-22. doi: 10.1016/j.mce.2008.09.005. Epub 2008 Sep 17. Review. PubMed [citation] PMID: 18838102, PMCID: PMC2662347*

136. *Veldhuis JD. Changes in pituitary function with ageing and implications for patient care. Nat Rev Endocrinol. 2013 Apr;9(4):205-15. doi: 10.1038/ nrendo.2013.38. Epub 2013 Feb 26. Review. PubMed [citation] PMID: 23438832, PMCID: PMC3920108*

137. *Veldhuis JD, Erickson D, Iranmanesh A, Miles JM, Bowers CY. Sex-steroid control of the aging somatotropic axis. Endocrinol Metab Clin North Am. 2005 Dec;34(4):877-93, viii. Review. No abstract available. PubMed [citation] PMID: 16310628*

138. *Vermeulen A. Ageing, hormones, body composition, metabolic effects. World J Urol. 2002 May;20(1):23-7. Review. PubMed [citation] PMID: 12088185*

139. *Vermeulen A. Andropause. Maturitas. 2000 Jan 15;34(1):5-15. Review. PubMed [citation] PMID: 10687877*

140. *Waddington KE, Jury EC. Manipulating membrane lipid profiles to restore T-cell function in autoimmunity. Biochem Soc Trans. 2015 Aug;43(4):745-51. doi: 10.1042/BST20150111. Epub 2015 Aug 3. PubMed [citation] PMID: 26551723*

141. *Wang M, Tan Y, Shi Y, Wang X, Liao Z, Wei P. Diabetes and Sarcopenic Obesity: Pathogenesis, Diagnosis, and Treatments. Front Endocrinol (Lausanne). 2020 Aug 25;11:568. doi: 10.3389/fendo.2020.00568. eCollection 2020. Review. PubMed [citation] PMID: 32982969, PMCID: PMC7477770*

142. *Weitzman ED. Circadian rhythms and episodic hormone secretion in man. Annu Rev Med. 1976;27:225-43. Review. No abstract available. PubMed [citation] PMID: 180872*

143. *Wilkinson CW, Peskind ER, Raskind MA. Decreased hypothalamic-pituitary-adrenal axis sensitivity to cortisol feedback inhibition in human aging. Neuroendocrinology. 1997 Jan;65(1):79-90. PubMed [citation] PMID: 9032777*

144. *Woods NF, Mitchell ES. Perimenopause: an update. Nurs Clin North Am. 2004 Mar;39(1):117-29. Review. PubMed [citation] PMID: 15062731*

145. *Wren AM. Gut and hormones and obesity. Front Horm Res.*

2008;36:165-181. doi: 10.1159/000115364. Review. PubMed [citation] PMID: 18230902

146. Yang Q, Alemany R, Casas J, Kitajka K, Lanier SM, Escribá PV. Influence of the membrane lipid structure on signal processing via G protein-coupled receptors. Mol Pharmacol. 2005 Jul;68(1):210-7. Epub 2005 Apr 18. PubMed [citation] PMID: 15837842

147. Yeap BB. Testosterone and ill-health in aging men. Nat Clin Pract Endocrinol Metab. 2009 Feb;5(2):113-21. doi: 10.1038/ncpendmet1050. Review. PubMed [citation] PMID: 19165223

148. Yerevanian A, Soukas AA. Metformin: Mechanisms in Human Obesity and Weight Loss. Curr Obes Rep. 2019 Jun;8(2):156-164. doi: 10.1007/ s13679-019-00335-3. Review. PubMed [citation] PMID: 30874963, PMCID: PMC6520185

149. Zhu S, Tian Z, Torigoe D, Zhao J, Xie P, Sugizaki T, Sato M, Horiguchi H, Terada K, Kadomatsu T, Miyata K, Oike Y. Aging- and obesity-related peri-muscular adipose tissue accelerates muscle atrophy. PLoS One. 2019 Aug 23;14(8):e0221366. doi: 10.1371/journal.pone.0221366. eCollection 2019. PubMed [citation] PMID: 31442231, PMCID: PMC6707561

150. The 4-Celled Tetrabaena socialis Nuclear Genome Reveals the Essential Components for Genetic Control of Cell Number at the Origin of Multicellularity in the Volvocine Lineage Jonathan Featherston, Yoko Arakaki, Erik R Hanschen, Patrick J Ferris, Richard E Michod, Bradley J S C Olson, Hisayoshi Nozaki, Pierre M DurandMolecular Biology and Evolution, Volume 35, Issue 4, April 2018, Pages 855–870, https://doi.org/10.1093/ molbev/msx332 Published:26 December 2017

151. В.М. Дильман "Большие Биологические Часы» (Введение в интегральную медицину). -М.: Знание, 1982 – 208 с. Ил.

152. Дильман, Владимир Михайлович "Эндокринологическая онкология: (Руководство для врачей). Л.: Медицина, 1983.- 408 с. ил

.

.

www.ingramcontent.com/pod-product-compliance
Lightning Source LLC
Chambersburg PA
CBHW022057020426
42335CB00012B/724